CONSUMER REPORTS

Health
Answer
Book

CONSUMER REPORTS

Health
Answer
Book

**The Editors of
Consumer Reports with**
JONATHAN LEFF

CONSUMER REPORTS BOOKS
A Division of Consumers Union
Yonkers, New York

Library of Congress Cataloging-in-Publication Data

Leff, Jonathan.
    Consumer Reports health answer book / the
editors of Consumer Reports with Jonathan Leff
        p. cm.
        Includes index.
        ISBN 0-89043-636-3
        1. Medicine, Popular—Miscellanea.   I. Consumer reports.
II. Title.
RC82.L45   1993
613—dc20   93-10613
                                                                  CIP

Design by GDS / Jeffrey L. Ward
First printing, September 1993
Manufactured in the United States of America

This book was printed on recycled paper. ♲

Consumer Reports Health Answer Book is a Consumer Reports Book published by Consumers Union, the nonprofit organization that publishes *Consumer Reports*, the monthly magazine of test reports, product Ratings, and buying guidance. Established in 1936, Consumers Union is chartered under the Not-for-Profit Corporation Law of the State of New York.

The purposes of Consumers Union, as stated in its charter, are to provide consumers with information and counsel on consumer goods and services, to give information on all matters relating to the expenditure of the family income, and to initiate and to cooperate with individual and group efforts seeking to create and maintain decent living standards.

Consumers Union derives its income solely from the sale of *Consumer Reports* and other publications. In addition, expenses of occasional public service efforts may be met, in part, by nonrestrictive, noncommercial contributions, grants, and fees. Consumers Union accepts no advertising or product samples and is not beholden in any way to any commercial interest. Its Ratings and reports are solely for the use of the readers of its publications. Neither the Ratings, nor the reports, nor any Consumers Union publications, including this book, may be used in advertising or for any commercial purpose. Consumers Union will take all steps open to it to prevent such uses of its material, its name, or the name of *Consumer Reports*.

Contents

CONSUMER REPORTS

Health
Answer
Book

Introduction

One of *Consumer Reports* popular features is "A Question of Health," a series of questions and answers on a wide variety of health topics. A popular column in *Consumer Reports on Health* newsletter is "On Your Mind." Most of the contents of *Consumer Reports Health Answer Book* have been drawn from these two sources. All of the information has been reviewed and updated by Consumers Union's medical consultants prior to publication in this book.

A number of the questions presented here reflect concern with health problems currently in the news: AIDS, recent developments in drugs and medications, the latest surgical techniques, cholesterol facts and figures, and controversial nutritional and diet data. But many questions are those you may always have wanted to ask your doctor at one time or another—about such common complaints as leg cramps, cold sores, skin lesions, itching, varicose veins, a runny nose, cold hands, and various aches and pains ranging from arthritis and shingles to toothache and burning feet.

Consumer Reports Health Answer Book also includes many of the "Office Visit" columns, a regular feature in *Consumer Reports on Health*, by Marvin M. Lipman, M.D., Consumers Union's chief medical adviser. These discussions, highly readable and full of practical advice, cover a wide range of health problems, including anemia, irritable bowel syndrome, bad breath, snoring, headaches, and hair loss, among others. The case histories are taken directly from Dr. Lipman's own medical practice.

Several of the "Office Visit" columns offer candid commentaries on how to improve communication with your doctor, including what to do if your physician is impatient, negligent, or just too busy to answer your phone calls. Irwin D. Mandel, D.D.S., Consumers Union's dental consultant, joins the discussion with an "Office Visit" that describes ways of evaluating your dentist and, if necessary, how to find a new one.

Consumer Reports Health Answer Book is easy to use. Each major topic is listed alphabetically, with specific problems arranged under the appropriate heading. Following many of the main questions and answers are "Office Visit" columns that discuss the same topic from a different angle and in greater detail.

This book includes frequent references to drugs, both prescription and over-the-counter. For ease of identification, prescription drugs are listed by generic name, followed in parentheses by a sampling of brand names for that particular drug. Such references are not a comprehensive listing of all brands available, nor do they represent an endorsement of the drugs.

Simply check the table of contents or consult the index to find the subjects that interest you. You're bound to find some questions (and answers) or some health topic discussions that affect you, a family member, or a friend. Or read the book straight through. Once you get started, *Consumer Reports Health Answer Book* is hard to put down.

We think you'll find this book enlightening, entertaining, and a valuable source of reliable medical information.

AIDS and HIV

HIV-Positive or Not?

Q. *I'm 56 and have donated over 90 pints of blood over the years. After my last donation, I received a letter that read, in part: "Unfortunately, we can no longer accept you as a donor because there was something in your blood detected in our HIV antibody screening test. . . . However, we did additional testing by a more specific method, and the final result was negative for antibody to HIV. . . . It is our policy, based on current federal and state guidelines, not to accept blood donors whose blood has been found to be falsely positive for anti-HIV."*

What's going on?

A. Screening tests for HIV (human immunodeficiency virus, the cause of AIDS) work by detecting antibodies to the virus, also known as anti-HIV. The tests, designed for maximum sensitivity, are sometimes triggered by factors other than HIV antibodies—a "false-positive" result. You can have a false-positive test, for example, if you have had a recent flu shot.

The first screening test your blood bank used was probably the ELISA test, a quick, relatively cheap screening method that occasionally yields false-positive results. Blood that tests positive for HIV in the ELISA test is then put through a more specific and expensive test called the Western Blot. Even though the second test showed no HIV antibodies in your blood, the blood bank's rules required it to reject your blood—on the theoretical but extremely unlikely possibility that the first test could be right and the second one wrong.

To rule out such a possibility, speak to your doctor about risk factors and ask to be retested with a newer, "recombinant" screening test that is less likely to give a false-positive result. If that test is negative and you'd like to resume blood donations, see if the blood bank has a donor reentry program. You'll have to wait six months and then get negative results on both the ELISA and Western Blot tests before being allowed to donate.

☐ OFFICE VISIT

Testing for AIDS: A Personal Decision

Home from college for the holidays, a young man comes in for a checkup. I've known him since he was a boy. Over the years, I've helped him through the usual assortment of sore throats and sprains. Now he tells me he's worried about AIDS.

"I've thought about being tested," he says. "But I'm not sure I want to know. What good will it do me?"

It may seem pointless to test for an incurable, fatal disease. But there are good reasons to do so. Early detection of HIV (human immunodeficiency virus) means that a person is a candidate for AZT, a drug that can delay the deterioration of the immune system that eventually leads to AIDS. That delay may eventually allow the person to benefit from any medical advances that might take place. And recent scientific advances allow people who know early on that they're infected with HIV to take at least some steps to compensate for a decreased resistance to other diseases. Certain drugs, for example, can help protect against pneumocystis carinii pneumonia, the most common of the "opportunistic" infections that attack people who have AIDS. Vaccinations against influenza and pneumococcal pneumonia are helpful before the immune system has been extensively compromised.

Another reason someone infected with the virus should know as early as possible is so that he or she can change any behavior that's endangering others. Of course, that change can and should take place even without the knowledge of HIV positivity.

Assessing the Risk

Because these medical steps may prolong life and health, I encourage anyone who has reason to be concerned about AIDS to be tested. People whose behavior during the past 10 years or so places them at highest risk include:

- ☐ Gay or bisexual males—especially those with multiple partners, or who have had anal intercourse without a condom.
- ☐ Intravenous drug users who share syringes, needles, or other paraphernalia.
- ☐ Sexual partners of those people

Other persons whose behavior places them at moderate risk include those with multiple heterosexual contacts.

I would want to know whether my young patient's concern about AIDS is justified. Is he gay? Does he or his sexual partners inject drugs? How many sexual partners has he had? What precautions does he take against sexually transmitted diseases?

But I wonder if my patient trusts me, or any physician, enough to discuss these intimate subjects frankly. I review those risky behavior patterns with my patient, but I don't ask him to tell me more about himself than he wants to.

Ideally, all medical practitioners would deserve the trust of their patients and would protect their confidences. But bigotry and discrimination exist in medicine, as elsewhere. My patients may not want to share their secrets with me, no matter how closely I guard their privacy and how nonjudgmental I am. So, while I try to earn my patient's trust, I also let him know testing is available anonymously through most state health departments.

My advice on HIV testing is not as clear-cut as other medical advice I've given him over the years, but AIDS isn't like anything else we've ever faced. I tell him as much as I can, considering how little is known.

Now it's up to him. Unless he decides to be tested on the spot, I'll encourage him to take time to think about it. If he decides to be tested, I'll tell him what to expect. If he'd rather not be tested, then confronting the issue should remind him that he can decrease his own risk for AIDS.

Allergies

Allergy Shots

Q. *I've had chronic nasal congestion and figured it was due to an allergy. After skin tests confirmed my hunch, my ear, nose, and throat doctor started giving me desensitization shots. He said I'll need them for the rest of my life. Is that true?*

A. Probably not. Your allergic sensitivity may eventually fade. Allergy shots should be given only as frequently as needed to control symptoms. Typically, that means once a month for most of the year—perhaps more often during allergy season. If symptoms improve over time, the interval between shots can be increased.

Antihistamines in Advance?

Q. *Should antihistamines be taken prior to allergy season, before symptoms develop, in order to build up immunity against the onslaught of allergens?*

A. No. Antihistamines have no such "priming" effect. They help to combat allergic symptoms only when allergens (allergy-inducing substances) are present.

Most people can safely take antihistamines daily throughout the allergy season. However, in some people antihistamines can cause distressing side effects, including confusion, dizziness, drowsiness, urinary retention, and disturbed vision. Pregnant or breast-feeding women, men with prostate problems, and people with glaucoma should consult a physician before taking an antihistamine.

Two nonsedating antihistamines—terfenadine (*Seldane*) and astemizole (*Hismanal*)—are available by prescription. Aside from not causing drowsiness, their side effects are similar to over-the-counter antihistamines.

The Food and Drug Administration (FDA) has warned that extremely high blood levels of either drug can cause potentially fatal abnormal heart rhythms.

To avoid harm:

☐ Don't exceed the prescribed dosage.
☐ If you have a liver disorder, stay off terfenadine and astemizole altogether, since such disorders can slow the breakdown of the drugs and allow them to build up in the blood.
☐ Avoid both terfenadine and astemizole if you're taking the antifungal drug ketoconazole (*Nizoral*) or antibiotics in the erythromycin family, including erythromycin (*E-Mycin*), clarithromycin (*Biarin*), azithromycin (*Zithromax*), and troleandomycin (*Tao*). Those drugs can boost blood levels of terfenadine to dangerous levels.
☐ Avoid both drugs if you have had abnormal heart rhythms.

Alzheimer's Disease

Aluminum and Antacids

Q. *I've heard that aluminum might cause Alzheimer's disease and other problems, so I was surprised to see you mention aluminum hydroxide as a safe antacid.*

A. There's no scientific evidence that aluminum ingested from antacids or any other source contributes to Alzheimer's and other dementias.

People with normal kidney function excrete virtually all the aluminum absorbed into the body. But older people (who may have decreased kidney function) and people with known kidney disease tend to retain aluminum within the body. Although that's not been shown to cause any harm in these individuals, they should use aluminum antacids only on a physician's advice.

Aluminum can contribute to health problems in some persons. For instance, aluminum-related bone disease has occurred in kidney patients on long-term hemodialysis. As a result, dialysis fluids are now more rigorously purified, and physicians try to avoid aluminum compounds—or at least use smaller amounts—in treating kidney disease.

☐ OFFICE VISIT

Chronic Illness: Caring for the Caregiver

"I can't take it anymore," a 64-year-old woman called to tell me. "Either he goes or I go."

Her 80-year-old husband, who has Alzheimer's disease, had been especially hard to handle for the past year. Several times, he wandered away from home late at night until the police brought him back. The day before she called me, he started a kitchen fire when he tried to warm some food on the stove. (The food was on a paper plate.) He was hospitalized with second-degree burns to his hands and chest.

His wife had been taking care of him at home for five years. She had kept her part-time job for a while, but eventually she realized that she couldn't leave him alone on the days she went to work. So she quit her job and became a full-time caregiver.

Now she was frustrated, depressed, and desperate. With the help of a hospital social worker, she had her husband transferred to a nursing home. Three months later, he died there. Plagued by feelings of guilt for not taking him back into their home, his wife began seeing a psychotherapist.

The Stress of Caregiving

Apart from the harrowing details, this woman's story is far from unique. More than 7 million Americans care for a dependent aging person—usually a spouse or parent. The average caregiver is about 60 years old, and most are women.

Studies show that caregivers get sick more often than other people the same age and may be more vulnerable to serious illness. That's hardly surprising.

The physical demands are exhausting. For an older caregiver, lifting, bathing, and dressing a helpless adult can lead to sprains and strains, even falls and fractures. Then there's the stress of having limited finances and unlimited expenses. Worst of all may be the emotional stress of watching a loved one deteriorate physically and mentally.

Finding Help: Getting Started

Sooner or later, most caregivers realize they're going to need help. I think the best way to start tracking down resources is by talking to a social worker. You can find one at your local hospital, at the county or state agency on aging, or in local religious, charitable, or other nonprofit organizations. (Check the Yellow Pages under "Social Services" or "Human Services." Or call your department of health.)

The social worker can tell you where to find programs and groups that can help you care for your spouse or parent. Some agencies offer financial advice, assistance with tax and Medicare forms, and help in locating special-needs housing. They may also administer services that provide transportation and meals.

At first, all you may need is someone to step in for a while to give you some time off. There are two main sources of such help:

☐ In some areas, volunteers organized by religious, local government, or other community groups will visit your home and spell you for a few hours. Or they may help with shopping or provide transportation, perhaps to get the ailing person to a doctor's appointment or an exercise class.

❑ Adult day-care programs are run by various community organizations such as churches, synagogues, Ys, and hospitals. The programs may last part of each weekday, but some run the full day whereas others are limited to one morning or afternoon a week. They typically offer personal care, meals, recreational activities, and various therapies. Transportation is usually provided. Some programs are based on a sliding scale, depending on your income; others may even be free.

Full-Time Help

Caregivers who need more than an occasional hand may have to hire an aide to work in their home regularly. Such aides can bathe, dress, and feed the patient; they can perform unskilled nursing tasks such as giving medications; and they can shop, cook, and do light housekeeping.

To find an aide, you can either hire someone yourself or rely on a home health agency. Doing it yourself—through newspaper ads or on the recommendation of a friend, relative, social worker, or member of the clergy—allows you to interview candidates and check their references. It may also save you money, since you pay the aide directly rather than through an agency. But the search can take a lot of time and effort. And if the person you hire doesn't work out or fails to show up, you're stuck with no help.

Home health agencies spare you the search, and they'll supply an immediate replacement if the aide quits or doesn't come. Although agencies are supposed to screen potential aides and provide at least some training, standards may be lax. Asking around for a reputable agency can help. More important, don't hesitate to have the agency keep sending someone new until you find a person you like and trust. If the agency objects, try a different agency.

Having an aide in for a full, eight-hour day costs roughly $200. Medicaid may pay most of the cost, if you're eligible. Medicare ordinarily covers only skilled-nursing services.

People caring for a terminally ill patient should consider a hospice program, designed to ease the patient's pain and help both patient and caregiver cope with impending death. Such programs, usually set up at home, arrange for care from many different people—including a visiting nurse, social worker, home health aide, clergy, and volunteers—as well as medical equipment and drugs. Medicare-certified hospice care is generally covered for six months. The National Hospice Helpline, 800-658-8898, offers useful information on hospice locations.

At some point, it just may not be feasible to continue caring for a chronically ill or disabled loved one at home. Then you'll want to look into institutional care. The options range from residence centers for mobile patients who need limited assistance to nursing homes for bedbound patients who need continual medical and personal care.

You can get a list of licensed facilities from your agency on aging. Or get recommendations from friends or professionals. Visit several facilities and observe how the staff interacts with patients. Try to come during visiting hours, so you can ask residents and their family members how they like the place.

Take Care of Yourself

To be an effective caregiver, it's important to look after your own needs as well. Here are a few more ways to care for yourself while you're caring for another:

☐ *Don't be a martyr.* Let family members and even friends know that the burden is too much for one person and that you'd appreciate their help from time to time.

☐ *Learn as much as you can* about the illness or disability of the person you're caring for so you'll know what to expect.

☐ *Join a caregiver support group.* In addition to providing emotional support, the group members can often steer you to reliable sources of help.

☐ *Take a vacation*—even if only for a few days. You can hire a home health aide to care for your loved one while you're gone. And some nursing homes will offer "respite care": They will accept people for a short stay to give caregivers a break.

Anemia

▭ OFFICE VISIT

Anemia: Do You Have Iron-Poor Blood?

My patient, a 37-year-old teacher, complained of feeling tired and listless for the past six months. Her menstrual periods had been heavier than usual for some time, and she'd heard that extra menstrual blood loss could lead to iron deficiency and cause fatigue. On the advice of a friend, she started taking a vitamin supplement containing iron. But her fatigue got worse.

Blood tests showed that she was indeed anemic due to iron deficiency. But although her heavy periods may have compounded the anemia, analysis of her stools showed that she was also losing blood from her bowel. The cause: an intestinal polyp.

After the polyp was removed, I started her on iron therapy at about 20 times the amount contained in the supplement she'd been taking. Over the next two months, her blood count slowly rose to normal.

By treating "iron poor" blood herself, my patient delayed diagnosis of that polyp, which might have been cancerous.

What Causes Anemia

Anemia simply means that there are fewer oxygen-carrying red blood cells in the bloodstream than is normal. This common condition is not a disease but a warning sign. If you treat just the sign, the underlying disorder can progress unchecked.

In some cases, red blood cells are scarce because the bone marrow isn't producing enough or because too many are being destroyed in the bloodstream or the spleen. But by far the most common cause of anemia is a deficiency of iron, a key component of red blood cells. And the most common cause of iron deficiency is not a lack of iron in the diet but bleeding—usually slow, chronic blood loss because of intestinal polyps, ulcers, fibroid tumors of the uterus, or even cancer. Chronic bleeding can also be caused by the regular use of aspirin, ibuprofen (*Advil, Nuprin*), or other nonsteroidal anti-inflammatory drugs.

Iron in the Diet

Iron-deficiency anemia can also stem from too little iron in the diet. But that's relatively uncommon in this country, except among some vegetarians and certain women.

Strict vegetarians should be particularly careful to get enough dietary iron, since the form found in plants is much less readily absorbed than that in meats. Whole grains and fiber can further reduce iron absorption. Nonmeat foods with the highest amounts of absorbable iron include dried fruits, legumes, and iron-fortified breads and cereals.

Pregnant women, including those who eat meat, should take a daily supplement containing 30 milligrams of iron to provide the extra iron needed to nourish a developing fetus. Some women who menstruate heavily may also need to take supplements to replace iron—but they should make sure that menstruation is the sole cause of their anemia before they start popping pills.

It's not a good idea to diagnose and treat "iron-poor blood" yourself, for the following reasons:

- ☐ There's far too little iron in a typical multivitamin pill to correct iron-deficiency anemia. Meanwhile, taking such a supplement could make you think you don't need to see a doctor.
- ☐ Taking iron supplements can also delay a diagnosis, because the stool turns black; that can mask the main warning sign of gastrointestinal bleeding.
- ☐ Iron preparations, available over the counter, contain up to seven times more iron than a multivitamin pill does. But you should consult your doctor to determine the proper dose. If you're susceptible to iron overloading and don't really have anemia, the extra iron can cause serious problems, such as damage to the liver, pancreas, and heart.

Arthritis, Joint, and Muscle Disorders

Arthritis and Cod-Liver Oil

Q. *I read in the book* Arthritis and Common Sense *that cod-liver oil can help treat arthritis. Can it really?*

A. No. The late author of that popular book, Dale Alexander— sometimes called "the Codfather"—claimed that the basic cause of arthritis is dry joints and that dietary oils, particularly cod-liver oil, relieve arthritis by lubricating the joints. That may have seemed like common sense to Alexander, but it's wrong.

There's never any "oil" in the joints, regardless of what you eat; the lubricating fluid, which resembles blood plasma, is secreted by the tissue lining the joints. Only in the Land of Oz can the joints be oiled. (For more on the mistreatment of arthritis, see *Health Schemes, Scams, and Frauds,* from Consumer Reports Books.)

Arthritis and Heart Attack

Q. *To treat my arthritis, I take* Trilisate, *which my doctor says is in the aspirin family. Since aspirin can help prevent heart attack, would the drug I'm taking offer some protection as well?*

A. No. Aspirin is believed to cut the risk of heart attack by making the blood less likely to clot. *Trilisate* (choline and magnesium salicylates) has no such effect. While other nonsteroidal anti-inflammatory drugs—such as ibuprofen (*Advil, Nuprin*), naproxen (*Naprosyn*), and piroxicam (*Feldene*)—can inhibit clotting somewhat, their blood-thinning effect is far less pronounced than that of aspirin. And only aspirin has been shown to reduce the risk of heart attack. (The other drugs, however, have not been adequately studied for this effect.)

Bursitis of the Hip

Q. *How common is bursitis of the hip, and what can be done about it? I had my first siege 10 months ago, and although* Feldene *helped a lot, the bursitis has not disappeared entirely.*

A. Although bursitis most often affects the shoulder, bursitis of the hip is still quite common. Knees and elbows are also vulnerable. At all these joints, tiny sacs called bursae are located between the tendon and bone. When a bursa becomes inflamed, often caused by injury or overuse, the joint aches. Standard treatment consists of rest and oral anti-inflammatory medication such as piroxicam *(Feldene)*. Sometimes injections of a corticosteroid drug directly into the bursa can be helpful. The inflammation and pain usually pass with time but can recur. In rare instances, surgery may be necessary.

Calcium Deposits

Q. *I have calcium deposits on the tendons in my shoulder. My doctor has prescribed anti-inflammatory drugs and tells me the deposits can be removed only by surgery. Is there any alternative? I also wonder if taking calcium supplements affects the condition.*

A. Calcium deposits tend to form on a tendon that's been inflamed for some time. Such deposits have nothing to do with the calcium you ingest, either in foods or in supplements. Anti-inflammatory drugs can relieve the discomfort temporarily. Graduated exercises, heat or cold treatments, and sometimes corticosteroid injections can also help. Surgery is usually reserved for severe cases, such as a "frozen" shoulder that doesn't respond to exercise therapy.

Cracked Knuckles

Q. *I have a habit of cracking my knuckles. Is that really harmful?*

A. The answer's still not certain. One recent study found that habitual knuckle crackers are more likely to have swollen hands and a weaker grip. The researchers concluded that the habit "results in functional hand impairment." But it's also possible that such impairment simply results from the loose joints that allow people to crack their knuckles in the first place. To play it safe, it's probably best to heed your mother's advice and stop cracking your knuckles.

Fibromyositis: What Does It Mean?

Q. *I have been diagnosed as having fibromyositis, which comes and goes. I would appreciate an explanation of what it is and whether it is curable or controllable.*

A. Fibromyositis, also known as fibrositis or fibromyalgia, refers to a disorder of unknown cause that is characterized by recurrent pain in the joints, muscles, or tendons. Often small, specific areas called "trigger points" are tender to the touch. Physical strain and cold or damp weather can make the disorder worse. Frequently, the pain is associated with other symptoms, such as insomnia, fatigue, or anxiety. Laboratory tests are usually normal. There are several treatments: physiotherapy, warm or cold compresses, anti-inflammatory medication, and sometimes anesthetic or cortisone injected directly into the trigger points. The symptoms fade fairly rapidly for some people; for others, the disorder can last for years.

Gold for Arthritis

Q. *For the past six months, I've had weekly injections of gold, which have helped my rheumatoid arthritis. Now my physician has recommended a maintenance injection every four or five weeks for the rest of my life. What are the long-range risks?*

A. Mainly skin rashes, mouth ulcers, and damage to the kidneys or bone marrow, where blood cells are manufactured. Any side effects of gold injections will usually develop during the first few months of treatment, but they can surface during the maintenance period as well. So you'll need a blood count and urine test before each injection.

A possible alternative is auranofin (*Ridaura*), an oral gold preparation. Whereas some of the injectable's side effects may be less common with the oral form, the latter carries its own possible side effects and may not be as effective.

Gout and the Diet

Q. *In addition to taking medication for gout, I also avoid foods high in purine—such as animal organs, herring, mushrooms, sardines, and spinach. I've been told my list of purine-containing foods is incomplete. What others should I avoid?*

A. Many other foods contain purines, notably anchovies, goose, mussels, scallops, yeast, and meat derivatives such as soup stock and gravy. But avoiding purine-containing foods may not be as necessary as it once was.

Gout is a heritable disease marked by an excess of uric acid in the blood. Severe dietary restriction for people with gout can indeed decrease blood levels of uric acid somewhat. However, today's medications, including allopurinol (*Lopurin, Zyloprim*) and probenecid (*Benemid, Probalan*), can do the job much better. So, moderation in diet rather than avoidance of certain foods is sufficient for most people with gout.

Alcohol, however, is one dietary item that should be restricted, since it may trigger an acute attack of gout.

Pseudo-Gout: What Is It?

Q. *A few months ago I came down with an ailment the medical people refer to as pseudo-gout. What in the world do I have?*

A. You have an illness known as chondrocalcinosis, characterized by painful, stiff joints caused by the buildup of calcium salts in the cartilage. Much less common than regular gout, pseudo-gout affects both men and women equally (gout affects mostly men) and causes attacks of pain that can be less predictable than those of gout. Like gout, pseudo-gout has no cure. Acute attacks can be controlled by colchicine—an anti-inflammatory drug that is specific for gout and pseudo-gout—or by using another anti-inflammatory drug such as ibuprofen. The latter can also be used in long-term maintenance for those afflicted with repeat episodes.

Muscle Cramps

Q. *As I've grown older, I've started getting muscle cramps. What can I do about them?*

A. For most cramps, stretch. If a spasm strikes the calf (by far the most common cramp site), pull the front of the foot up toward the knee. Since cramps usually result from muscle fatigue, you may be able to prevent such spasms by gently stretching before you exercise your calves. Stand a few feet from a wall, brace yourself against the wall with your hands, and lean forward, keeping your heels on the ground until you feel a pull in your calves. This maneuver before bedtime can also help prevent unexplained nighttime spasms.

If the cause isn't muscle fatigue, your physician may find other, possibly treatable causes. These can include circulatory problems, hyperventilation, an underactive thyroid, and low blood levels of calcium or (rarely) magnesium. If there's no underlying problem and stretching doesn't help, your physician might prescribe quinine.

Potatoes and Arthritis

Q. *Is it true that toxins in potatoes and other plants of the nightshade family—including tomatoes, peppers, and eggplant—can exacerbate or even cause arthritis in some people?*

A. There's no scientific evidence to support that old folk legend. If it were true, populations that eat lots of potatoes would presumably have a higher incidence of arthritis. Epidemiological studies have shown that they don't.

Restless Legs

Q. *During the evening or at night, when I'm in bed, I'm often unable to hold my legs still. What could be the matter?*

A. You probably have restless legs syndrome, in which an aching or crawling sensation in the leg muscles forces you to move your legs. Getting up and walking around tends to relieve the symptoms, but they usually recur when you return to bed. Restless legs may keep you from getting to sleep, but they'll seldom awaken you once you are asleep.

The cause of restless legs syndrome is unknown. Many treatments have been tried, including hot or cold packs, over-the-counter pain relievers, antihistamines, muscle relaxants, and sleeping potions. None has been shown to work consistently.

Rub It In

Q. *What is it about* Eucalyptamint *that relieves the pain of arthritis?*

A. Paradoxically, *Eucalyptamint*, like other muscle-ache and arthritis rubs, provides relief by acting as a counterirritant. Rubbed into the skin, it produces a mild local inflammation that crowds out pain messages from nearby muscles and joints. Arthritis rubs also create heat by increasing blood flow to the area; because of the risk of a burn, they should never be used together with a heating pad.

Tetracycline and Arthritis

Q. *Can tetracycline help people with rheumatoid arthritis?*

A. The only evidence that tetracycline fights rheumatoid arthritis comes from a few poorly designed studies. Another antibiotic, sulfasalazine (*Azulfidine*), has shown promise for people who have clinical signs of rheumatoid arthritis but a negative blood test.

Asthma and Lung Problems

Blood Clots in the Lung

Q. *Four weeks after a hysterectomy, my 62-year-old mother died suddenly due to pulmonary emboli, or blood clots in her lung. Should my sisters and I worry that this could happen to us after surgery?*

A. That depends. Susceptibility to pulmonary embolism, which generally develops only after surgery or prolonged bed rest, is not inherited directly. However, two risk factors for the condition—obesity and severe varicose veins—do run in families. Other risk factors include heart failure, certain cancers, and a history of phlebitis (inflamed veins).

People predisposed to pulmonary embolism may receive anticlotting medication after they've undergone abdominal, pelvic, or certain orthopedic operations—or if they'll be bedridden for a long time.

Alternatives to Steroids

Q. *I take oral steroids—5 milligrams of prednisone in the morning and 5 milligrams at night—for severe asthma. But I'm concerned about harmful effects and would prefer an alternative drug. What do you recommend?*

A. While oral steroids can be very effective in chronic asthma, their long-term use can cause side effects such as bone thinning, hypertension, and diabetes. Accordingly, before starting a patient on oral steroids, doctors prefer to treat chronic asthma with inhaled beta agonists (*Atupen, Proventil*), inhaled corticosteroids (*Aerobid, Azmacort*), or, in children, inhaled cromolyn (*Intal*) or oral theophylline. If you need an oral corticosteroid, you may mitigate side effects by taking the daily dose in the morning or—better still—every other day. But changing corticosteroid dosage is a tricky business and must be done under close medical supervision.

Good Moves for Asthmatics

Q. *I'm considering a change of climate to help relieve my asthma. I've heard that the dry air of the desert Southwest is beneficial, but also that salty sea air can help. Can you clear up this contradiction?*

A. The friendliest locale for asthma sufferers is one that's free of pollutants, airborne allergens, and frigid weather. Traditionally, people with asthma migrated to Arizona for its warm, dry climate, although the benefit came primarily from leaving behind industrial air pollution and high pollen counts. As Arizona cities have grown, however, the environment there has become less favorable for asthmatics.

Sea air has no effect on asthma.

Chest Congestion

Q. *I often have congestion in my nose and ears but also in my chest. What over-the-counter drugs would you recommend to loosen this congestion in my chest so I can cough it up and spit it out?*

A. The only FDA-approved expectorant for loosening phlegm is guaifenesin. It's found in *Breonesin* tablets, plain *Robitussin* syrup, *Scot-tussin* syrup, and other over-the-counter products.

However, an expectorant doesn't address the underlying problem, and therefore should be used only occasionally. You seem to have a chronic problem in your sinuses or bronchial airways. You should be evaluated by a physician for allergies or any other problem that might be responsible for recurrent nasal and chest congestion.

☐ OFFICE VISIT

Emphysema Takes Smokers' Breath Away

Pausing frequently to cough, a 62-year-old accountant told me how difficult breathing had become. He took rapid, shallow breaths, taking longer to exhale than inhale. He tensed his neck muscles to help expand his chest as he inhaled and wheezed faintly as he exhaled. A chest X ray revealed that his lungs were overinflated. Blood tests showed abnormally low levels of oxygen and high levels of carbon dioxide.

"How much do you smoke?" I asked.

"Two packs a day since college," he said somewhat defiantly. "A couple of months ago, they banned smoking at the office. So I took early retirement."

My new patient was one of the more than 10 million Americans, nearly all of them over age 40, who suffer from chronic obstructive lung disease (COLD). In the United States, the disease limits the activity of more people than any other disorder and kills some 78,000 victims each year.

These grim figures are almost entirely a product of cigarette smoking. If no one smoked, the disease would be largely restricted to people with a rare genetic disorder. Other lung irritants, such as outdoor air pollution, can aggravate the symptoms of COLD. But they don't seem to cause the disease or accelerate its progress.

What Is COLD?

In chronic obstructive lung disease, less and less air flows in and out of the lungs. In the vast majority of cases, the disease is a combination of two related disorders: chronic bronchitis and emphysema.

Chronic bronchitis is a persistent inflammation of the branching tubes (bronchi) that carry air from the windpipe to the tiny sacs in the lungs. These air sacs are where the blood picks up oxygen and gets rid of carbon dioxide. The condition develops in virtually all cigarette smokers after about 10 years and is marked by a chronic, phlegm-producing cough. Thickening of the inflamed bronchial walls narrows the airways and causes wheezing and other breathing problems. Susceptibility to respiratory infections and lung cancer increases.

Emphysema tends to develop later than chronic bronchitis. The consequences may be more dire. In emphysema, the air sacs are progressively destroyed. Unable to expel air efficiently, the damaged lungs become overinflated. Carbon dioxide builds up in the blood, oxygen levels fall, and breathing grows increasingly difficult. The strain of pumping blood through the damaged lungs may weaken the heart. Eventually, the disease may lead to severe disability or death.

Although COLD is almost always caused by smoking, only 10 to 15 percent of smokers develop COLD. Researchers don't know why the disease strikes only certain smokers, nor can they identify susceptible individuals.

Quitting Can Save Your Life

The only way to prevent COLD is not to smoke. The best way to treat it is to quit smoking. In the early stages of the disease, quitting allows the swelling and excess mucus production in the bronchial tubes to subside. That tends to relieve the cough, as well as any wheezing or other difficulty breathing.

In the later stages of COLD, kicking the habit may no longer reverse the bronchial thickening. But quitting does slow the destruction of the air sacs in the lungs. That may prevent a minor problem from becoming serious or a serious problem from becoming fatal.

There are two other measures that may improve the chances of survival with COLD. Antibiotics can be given at the first sign of respiratory infection. And oxygen can be administered around the clock, at home, to patients with severe oxygen deficiency. (The oxygen flows into the patient's nose through a tube connected to a portable or stationary tank.)

An Unexpected Transformation

I asked my patient if he realized how much harm cigarette smoking had caused him.

"Sure I do," he said. "But there's no point in quitting now. The damage is done."

"There's more to come if you keep smoking," I told him. "You'll end up on a breathing machine, and eventually the disease will kill you."

I prescribed an aerosol bronchodilator to relax the muscles in the walls of the bronchial tubes. And I sent him to a registered respiratory therapist to learn breathing techniques and start an exercise conditioning program.

A month later, he returned with good news. He was wheezing less and breathing more easily. More important, he had stopped smoking.

☐ Back Pain

Disk Decision

Q. *Because of a herniated disk, I've been suffering from lower-back pain that radiates to my leg. Is surgery usually necessary, or could other treatment relieve the pain?*

A. Conservative treatment, including bed rest, physical therapy, anti-inflammatory drugs, and traction, is often successful in relieving pain from a herniated, or "slipped," disk. Unless the pain or numbness is severe or nerve function is impaired to the point of weakness of your leg muscles, you should try those alternatives for two to three months before resorting to surgery.

Bladder and Urinary Problems

Cancerous Bladder Polyps

Q. *My urologist found bladder polyps when he did a cystoscopy on me. After removing them, he said they were cancerous but "low-grade, superficial, and noninvasive." What causes malignant bladder polyps?*

A. Occasionally, a specific carcinogen can be pinpointed as the cause of malignant polyps. The main culprits are cigarette smoking and occupational exposure to aromatic amines, compounds used in many manufacturing and chemical processes. In most cases, however, there's no identifiable cause.

Malignant bladder polyps range from slow-growing, noninvasive tumors to aggressive cancers that rapidly invade the bladder wall. Bladder polyps can also turn out to be benign. In either case, the most effective treatment is removal of the polyps through a cystoscope, a lighted tube inserted into the bladder. After removal of a malignant polyp, the bladder should be reinspected cystoscopically every three to six months for several years. A chemical can also be instilled directly into the bladder to inhibit the development of additional polyps.

Interstitial Cystitis

Q. *What can you tell me about interstitial cystitis? I know it resembles a urinary-tract infection, but it's not an infection.*

A. You're right. Interstitial cystitis is a bladder inflammation, but infection is not to blame. Like a urinary-tract infection, the disease can provoke frequent, urgent urination. Unlike an infection, it often causes pain that is actually relieved by urination.

No one knows what causes interstitial cystitis, and diagnosis can be difficult. There is no cure, so treatment focuses on symptoms. Many approaches have been tried, including distending the bladder with fluid; infusing the bladder with a chemical called DMSO (*Rimso*); and giving oral medications such as pentosan polysulfate sodium (*Elmiran*), the antidepressant amitriptyline (*Elavil*), and various muscle relaxants for the bladder. None has worked consistently.

In a recent study, patients who didn't have severe pain gradually stretched their bladder by resisting the urge to urinate frequently. Each month, they increased the interval between trips to the bathroom by 15 to 30 minutes. After three months, 15 of the 21 patients reported at least a 50 percent reduction in the urgency and frequency of urination.

Since the disorder often defies medical therapy, patients have formed a self-help group: The Interstitial Cystitis Association (212–979–6057).

Long-Term Diuretics

Q. *I take a diuretic medication every day. Does the drug lose its effectiveness or cause any harm when taken for many years?*

A. No. Diuretics (drugs that increase urine output) are an effective long-term therapy for hypertension and other disorders. And unlike some drugs used for chronic conditions, diuretics don't damage the kidneys, liver, or other organs.

Does PPA Slow Urination?

Q. *Phenylpropanolamine seems to interfere with my urine flow. This misled two physicians into thinking I had a prostate problem. But I discovered, quite by accident, that the drug appears to be the problem. Is this possible?*

A. Yes. Phenylpropanolamine (PPA) is an oral decongestant combined with an antihistamine in products (such as *Dimetapp* and *Triaminic*) touted for the common cold. It's also the active ingredient in all over-the-counter diet pills. The side effects of PPA include elevation of blood pressure and rapid or irregular heartbeat and urinary retention. Some physicians prescribe PPA as a treatment for urinary incontinence.

Restless Nights

Q. *For the past couple of years, an aching fullness in my bladder has prompted me to get up as many as three to four times a night to urinate. I do not experience the same problem during the day. I am 25 years old, female, and otherwise in good health. Do I need to see a doctor?*

A. Not necessarily. First, try drinking less fluid with dinner and during the evening. In particular, refrain from alcohol, which is a diuretic and can cause frequent urination. But if these simple measures don't work, see your doctor. Your "nocturia" could be due to an enlarged pelvic structure pressing on the bladder when you lie down, the nighttime release of daytime water retention, or a kidney disorder.

Blood Pressure

Diuretics in the Desert

Q. *My sister's physician put her on a daily diuretic to treat hypertension. She'll be taking a trip to the desert soon. Should she use salt tablets to prevent dehydration?*

A. No. If the diuretic isn't causing excessive water loss now, dehydration from the heat shouldn't be a problem. Salt tablets might make the body retain water, but that's exactly what the diuretic is supposed to prevent. Your sister should just drink plenty of water to replace what she sweats away.

Heat and Blood Pressure

Q. Does using a Jacuzzi or sauna elevate blood pressure in people who already have hypertension?

A. No. In fact, high ambient temperature typically causes blood pressure to drop as blood vessels dilate in order to keep body temperature constant. That drop in blood pressure can cause you to faint, especially if you're already taking antihypertensive medication.

Low Blood Pressure

Q. Recently I tried to donate blood for the first time and was turned away because my blood pressure was too low (80 over 60 that morning). I'm 52 years old and, as far as I know, in good health. I eat a balanced diet and I exercise almost every day. But my blood pressure is usually only about 100 over 70. Should I be worried about that low level?

A. On the contrary, you should ask for a rebate on your life insurance premium! If you feel healthy, having a relatively low blood pressure like yours is good for the cardiovascular system, since it puts less stress on the blood vessels. If you were not in such good health, low blood pressure could indicate a disorder such as coronary heart disease or low blood volume due to blood loss. The only reason why low pressure would disqualify you as a donor is that the additional lowering due to losing a pint of blood could conceivably cause a fainting spell.

Safe with Normal Blood Pressure?

Q. *I'm 63 years old and in fine health as far as I know. For years my blood pressure has been in the neighborhood of 118/85, which I understand is quite good. If my blood pressure stays down, am I unlikely to experience a heart attack or stroke?*

A. Normal blood pressure is definitely an advantage, but it won't protect you completely. High blood pressure is only one of several risk factors for cardiovascular disease. Others include smoking, high blood cholesterol, lack of exercise, heredity, and diabetes. Nevertheless, recent studies have suggested that even mild elevations of blood pressure increase your risk of problems. That's why it's important to keep track of your pressure, even if it hasn't been high to date.

The Other Hypertension

Q. *What would cause an increase in a 70-year-old's systolic, or upper, blood-pressure reading while the diastolic pressure remains normal? How serious a problem is this?*

A. The stiffening of the arteries that typically occurs with advancing age can cause systolic blood pressure (the pressure in the arteries when the heart contracts) to rise above normal without affecting diastolic pressure (the pressure between contractions). An overactive thyroid or anemia can often produce the same effect. Temporary systolic blood-pressure hikes may result from exercise, stress, or excitement.

Unless extreme, increases in systolic blood pressure probably pose less risk than diastolic hypertension. Many doctors believe borderline systolic hypertension does not require treatment. Elevations above 160 mm/Hg, however, should be considered for treatment with a modified diet or with low-dose antihypertensive medication.

Calcium

Aspirin and Kidney Stones?

Q. *During the last 50 years, I've had six kidney-stone attacks. The last one was about 10 years ago. One doctor told me that I had too much calcium in my system. I've heard that aspirin adds to my calcium levels and thus increases my chance of having another kidney-stone attack. Is that true?*

A. No. Aspirin itself doesn't affect the level of calcium in your blood or urine. Even aspirin buffered with calcium carbonate (*Ascriptin, Bufferin, Magnaprin*) doesn't contain enough calcium to affect those levels significantly.

Kidney Stones and Calcium

Q. *My 27-year-old daughter has had surgery twice for kidney stones. Her doctor told her to eliminate high-calcium foods from her diet. My concern is that a low-calcium diet will put her at high risk for osteoporosis. Would you comment?*

A. A low-calcium diet can increase the risk of osteoporosis, an abnormal loss of bone that can lead to fractures in later years. Your daughter's chances of avoiding osteoporosis will improve if she exercises regularly, doesn't smoke, and avoids heavy intake of alcohol and caffeine. There is now evidence that low-calcium diets can actually increase the frequency of kidney stones whereas high-calcium diets can do the opposite. This seeming paradox may have to do with the effect of dietary calcium on oxalates in the intestine.

Tums for the Bones

Q. My doctor told me to take Tums, which is calcium carbonate, as an inexpensive alternative to calcium pills. However, the bottle warns against taking the maximum dose for more than two weeks. Is it safe to take Tums indefinitely?

A. Yes, if you're just taking the modest dose needed as a supplement. Adults should get about 1,000 milligrams of calcium daily, which frequently can be obtained from food alone; postmenopausal women are often advised to obtain as much as 1,000 to 1,500 milligrams a day from food and supplements. Regular Tums provides 200 milligrams of calcium per tablet.

The warning on the Tums bottle refers to its use as an antacid: Prolonged need for antacids should be evaluated by a doctor. Moreover, large amounts of calcium—such as the maximum dose of 16 tablets a day for indigestion—can cause constipation, abdominal pain, and kidney stones if taken over a long period.

Calcium in Tums

Q. You told a reader that taking four Tums a day as a calcium supplement was "fine." I've read that the body doesn't absorb the calcium carbonate in Tums well. Isn't there a more absorbable calcium supplement?

A. Actually, calcium carbonate is readily absorbed—especially from Tums. On average, 40 percent of the elemental calcium in Tums reaches the bloodstream. (Elemental calcium refers to the calcium itself, as opposed to the entire calcium-carbonate compound.) With other calcium-carbonate supplements, such as BioCal, Os-Cal, and Rolaids Calcium Rich, about 30 percent is absorbed. That's still quite good: About 30 to 35 percent of the calcium in milk is absorbed.

Tums for Calcium?

Q. *My doctor suggested I take four* Tums *tablets a day to add calcium to my diet. In your antacid report, you warned that prolonged use of calcium carbonate can actually promote heartburn as well as lead to dependency on the drug relief. Should I stop taking* Tums?

A. Not if it isn't causing a problem. Although antacids containing calcium carbonate can lead to acid rebound by stimulating the secretion of stomach acid, this effect depends on the dose. If you can consume four tablets a day without suffering heartburn, fine.

Calcium Absorption

Q. *I have osteoporosis and need to take supplemental calcium. I also eat lots of whole grains, but recently I've read that the phytic acid in them interferes with the absorption of calcium. Is that true?*

A. Yes. Moreover, calcium supplements themselves can interfere with the absorption of other nutrients in foods. So take your calcium with water at bedtime.

Calcium After 35

Q. *Is it true that your calcium intake doesn't matter after age 35 or so?*

A. No. Bone density in both men and women begins to decline gradually at about age 35. To forestall bone loss, all adults should get at least 1,000 milligrams of calcium daily. But in some women after menopause, bone density plummets for several years. The National Institutes of Health recommends an extra 500 milligrams for postmenopausal women who are at high risk of developing osteoporosis (weakened bones) and who are not on estrogen replacement therapy. Risk factors for osteoporosis include early menopause (either natural or surgically induced), a mother or sister with severe osteoporosis, white or Asian background, sedentary life-style, smoking, heavy drinking, and a low daily consumption of calcium (fewer than 1,000 milligrams) prior to menopause.

Calcium and Bloating

Q. *I take 1,000 milligrams of* Os-Cal *every day. Could that calcium supplement be contributing to my abdominal bloating?*

A. It's possible. Calcium carbonate, the compound in Os-Cal and many other calcium supplements, can cause constipation, which, in turn, can cause bloating. Other forms of calcium may be less constipating: calcium citrate, calcium gluconate, and calcium lactate. You might try switching to one of those forms. However, they do contain less calcium, so you'd have to take more to get an amount equal to that supplied by calcium carbonate. (Compare the labels for elemental calcium content—the amount of calcium itself as opposed to the entire calcium compound.)

Calcium and Lactose

Q. *I'm a 33-year-old man who can't digest lactose. Since I can't drink milk, I'm concerned that I don't get enough calcium in my diet. So I take a 500-milligram supplement twice a day. Is that necessary?*

A. It's a good idea to get 1,000 milligrams of calcium every day, but you can get that without supplements. One way is to consume milk products with the help of *Lactaid*, which contains the digestive enzyme lactase. Or you could drink a lactose-reduced milk. Buttermilk and yogurt probably wouldn't trouble you either. Nondairy sources of calcium include broccoli, greens (except spinach), kale, legumes (dried beans, peas, and lentils), and canned sardines and salmon.

Magnesium and Calcium

Q. *I was surprised that you didn't mention magnesium in your recent report on calcium. Doesn't magnesium help the body absorb calcium?*

A. No. Magnesium has nothing to do with calcium absorption. The only nutrient that's known to help the body absorb calcium is vitamin D, and adequate sun exposure plus dietary sources provides plenty.

☐ Cardiovascular Disorders

Accurate Angiogram

Q. *Before I started a strenuous exercise program, my doctor ordered an exercise stress test to check my heart, even though I have no symptoms of coronary heart disease. That test was inconclusive, so I had a thallium stress test, which indicated some coronary disease. To confirm that finding, I underwent angiography, which found no sign of disease. Which test should I believe?*

A. Angiography. This procedure, in which the coronary arteries are injected with dye and examined by X ray, is the most accurate test for blocked coronary arteries. The two stress tests are safer and less expensive than angiography, which is why they're generally done first. However, it is possible for those stress tests to turn up positive when there's actually nothing wrong.

Aspirin, TIA, and Ulcers

Q. *Several years ago, I experienced a transient ischemic attack (TIA), which my physician said indicates a risk of stroke. As a precaution, he recommended aspirin therapy to reduce the chance of blood clots. After an episode of stomach bleeding, attributed to aspirin's effect on a possible ulcer condition, I turned to Ecotrin, a coated aspirin. Should I stop using any kind of aspirin?*

A. Probably not. Aspirin coated with an acid-resistant shell (*Ecotrin* and generic versions) should dissolve after leaving the stomach and thus cause less irritation than uncoated aspirin. It offers the anticlotting benefits of aspirin, with less gastrointestinal risk. These benefits are important after a TIA, in which blood flow to the brain is temporarily interrupted.

But considering your history of gastrointestinal bleeding from aspirin, you should have blood counts every couple of months. You can also visually check your stool for signs of internal bleeding (which turns the stool black).

For ordinary pain relief, people with a history of ulcers are better off taking acetaminophen.

Atypical Angina?

Q. *I've read that angina, the type of chest pain that signals coronary heart disease, is usually brought on by exercise and relieved by rest. I sometimes experience chest discomfort while I'm resting but never while I'm exercising. Could that discomfort still be angina?*

A. It's unlikely. But an uncommon form of coronary disease can cause angina when you're resting or asleep—due to arterial spasm, not blockage. To rule out that possibility, your physician could have you wear a heart monitor for 24 hours. You should also have a treadmill exercise test, even though you haven't noticed the pain while exercising.

If these tests find no sign of coronary disease, your physician will investigate other possible causes of your discomfort. It's most likely to be a temporary problem, such as heartburn or muscle spasms. Occasionally, however, the discomfort reflects a chronic disorder, such as hiatal hernia or gallbladder disease.

Blocked Bundle Branch

Q. I'm a 50-year-old male with a "right bundle branch block." Is that cause for concern?

A. Not necessarily. The bundle branches are fibers within the heart muscle that transmit nerve impulses, causing the right and left ventricles to contract and pump blood into the arteries. Occasionally, transmission in one of the bundles becomes blocked, probably due to a clot in a tiny blood vessel feeding the bundle. The affected ventricle then contracts later than the other ventricle; this shows up as a characteristic pattern on an electrocardiogram. There are usually no symptoms, and there's no treatment.

A blocked bundle branch, particularly on the left, does increase the risk of subsequent heart attack somewhat. That risk is compounded by the presence of other risk factors for coronary heart disease: high blood-cholesterol levels, hypertension, male gender, diabetes, age, smoking, and a family history of coronary heart disease before age 55.

Generic Heart Drugs

Q. My cardiologist does not prescribe generic medications. As a result, I recently purchased brand-name drugs at four times the cost of generics. When I objected, he told me that generic cardiac medications vary significantly in quality. Do you care to comment?

A. In the 1970s, there were problems with generic versions of one heart medication, digoxin. Today, however, such problems no longer exist. Manufacturers of generic medications must prove that their drug is bioequivalent to the name brand—that is, that it is absorbed by the body at the same rate. To our knowledge, no study has shown a problem in efficacy with any generic cardiac medication that the FDA has deemed interchangeable with a name brand. In any case, if you are taking quinidine or other cardiac drugs—generic or not—your physician should periodically measure blood levels of the medication for safety and efficacy.

Heart Palpitations

Q. *I'm 62 and have had heart palpitations for years. What can you tell me about them?*

A. "Palpitations" is a nonmedical term for any heart rhythm that feels abnormal. That can include extra beats, dropped beats, forceful beats, rapid beats, or irregular beats. For proper diagnosis, the abnormality must first be "captured" on an electrocardiogram or on a 24-hour heartbeat recording. Palpitations can be caused by emotional stress, an overactive thyroid, certain medications, or diseases of the coronary arteries, heart muscle, or heart valves. Sometimes, there's no detectable cause.

At some point soon, you probably should have your palpitations checked, but first try eliminating a few things on your own—caffeine (coffee, tea, cocoa, chocolate, soda), nasal decongestants, appetite suppressants—and see if it makes a difference.

Magnesium and the Heart

Q. *What does a low level of magnesium have to do with abnormal heartbeats?*

A. Too little magnesium in the blood, an uncommon condition sometimes caused by chronic diarrhea or excessive alcohol intake, can lead to a type of abnormal heart rhythm known as tachyarrhythmia (rapid heartbeats). Supplemental magnesium can correct the problem. However, since too much magnesium can also adversely affect the heart, magnesium blood levels must be monitored closely.

Mitral Valve Prolapse

Q. *I am in my mid-thirties. A few years ago I was diagnosed as having a heart condition called mitral valve prolapse. What exactly is it, and does it make jogging risky?*

A. Mitral valve prolapse (MVP), which now appears to be more common than doctors previously realized, is usually a harmless condition. It involves a ballooning of the heart's mitral valve leaflets or flaps, which control blood flow between the left atrium and left ventricle. Physicians suspect MVP when they hear a certain type of heart murmur or a clicking sound through the stethoscope.

For the vast majority of people with MVP, the only health risk is a mitral valve infection following dental procedures that involve bleeding. If you have MVP, let your dentist know; antibiotics can eliminate the risk. As for exercise, most people with MVP can follow a sensible program. Ask your doctor.

Walking Test

Q. *The results of a recent walking test showed that, to qualify as moderately fit, a person over 60 must have a lower heart rate than a person of 20 walking at the same speed. Is this true?*

A. You read the test results correctly. When two people who take the test come out with the same heart rate, or pulse rate, the younger person is more fit. That's because younger people have a higher maximum heart rate—if necessary, their heart can beat faster and pump more blood than an older person's heart. So with identical heart rates, the younger person is always farther from his or her maximum rate, which means there's more cardiac capacity still in reserve. The older person would need a lower heart rate to have the same reserve capacity.

Warming Cold Hands

Q. *What causes cold hands, and what can I do about it?*

A. The most common cause, other than cold weather, is simple nervousness. When you're nervous, the surface capillaries in the hands and feet constrict, causing a feeling of coldness. There's not much you can do about that.

Less commonly, cold hands can reflect Raynaud's syndrome. When exposed to cold, the fingers or toes actually turn white. This change is caused by narrowing of the arteries that supply them. Medications such as nifedipine *(Procardia)* and prazocin *(Minipres)*, available by prescription, can help. Occasionally biofeedback techniques are useful.

Walk Away from Leg Pain

Q. *I suffer from leg pain because of poor circulation. You mentioned that it's possible to relieve the condition by exercising. What type of exercise do you suggest?*

A. Simply walking, typically for a total of a half hour to an hour per day. The most effective regimen involves walking to the point of pain, stopping and waiting for the pain to subside, and then starting up again. But check with your physician first to make sure that would be safe for you.

Esophageal Spasm

Q. *How can you tell chest pain caused by angina from that caused by a spasm of the esophagus?*

A. It's not always easy. Both types of pain are typically felt behind the breastbone. And the pain caused by an esophageal spasm often responds to nitroglycerin, the heart medication used to treat angina. However, there are three characteristics that do tend to set esophageal pain apart: (1) Unlike angina, it's more likely to occur when you're at rest; (2) it's often related to eating; and (3) it may be accompanied by difficulty in swallowing.

Since it can be difficult to tell the two disorders apart by symptoms alone, your physician may need to do some specific testing. Angina is usually evaluated by an exercise test (usually a treadmill test); esophageal spasm can be determined by a manometric test, in which you swallow a tube that measures esophageal muscle tension.

⬜ OFFICE VISIT

Chest Pain: The Heart of the Matter

The pain in my chest intensifies as I reach for a book on the shelf behind my desk. Inevitably, the fear of heart attack accompanies any chest pain.

But I remember last night's squash match and the lunge to make a point. The pain dulls as I drop my arm and returns when I lift it again. Making that shot apparently cost me a strained chest muscle.

Chest pain often has nothing to do with coronary disease. Most of my patients with chest pain have no cardiovascular problem at all. The cause of the chest pain is usually some minor, temporary problem—like my squash injury. In some cases, a serious, chronic condition other than coronary disease is responsible for chest pain.

Where Does It Hurt?

Patients who come to me with chest pain often have minor musculoskeletal problems. Unlike cardiac pain, pain from a strained chest muscle intensifies and subsides as the strained muscle fibers contract and relax when you move. This pain can last for days.

An injury to your ribs or breastbone can cause severe chest pain. You can usually identify such contusions and fractures because they're tender to the touch. Pain from a fractured rib can last for weeks. (Occasionally, arthritis affects one or more joints between the ribs and breastbone, causing chest pain.)

One of the most common sources of chest pain complaints is heartburn, a burning sensation beneath your breastbone that worsens when you lie down. Typically, stomach acid flows back into the lower part of the esophagus, resulting in painful inflammation of the esophageal lining. That reflux may be caused by a hiatal hernia (when a part of the stomach protrudes through the diaphragm) or by overindulgence at the dinner table.

Some people have chest pain as a result of muscle spasms in the esophagus. Spasms typically occur during or shortly after meals, causing painful pressure in the center of the chest. Swallowing becomes difficult, and saliva accumulates in the mouth. Despite these distinguishing features, pain from esophageal spasms is often mistaken for a symptom of coronary disease. The masquerade is made more convincing because the pain may be relieved by drugs often prescribed for cardiac pain.

If the chest pain is sharp and increases with breathing, the problem is likely to be pleurisy, which is an inflammation of the lining of the lungs often caused by pneumonia or a pulmonary embolism (blood clot to the lung). This pain is sometimes accompanied by fever and shortness of breath, and prompt medical care is vital.

One disorder that's especially difficult to distinguish from true coronary disease is pericarditis, an inflammation of the heart lining. This condition occurs most often in young adults and is usually caused by a viral infection accompanied by aches, chills, and fever.

Problems in other organs—some too far from the heart to seem likely suspects—occasionally lead to chest pain. Disorders of the gallbladder and pancreas can cause pain in the lower chest and upper abdomen. Gallbladder inflammation also causes pain near the right shoulder blade; pancreatic problems can bring on intense discomfort in the midback.

Chest pain—often with heart "palpitations" and sweating—may

be caused by emotional problems, especially severe anxiety and panic disorders.

When Pain Comes from the Heart

Despite the wide range of possible causes of chest pain, nearly everyone thinks first of heart attack and coronary disease. The classic symptom of coronary disease is angina pectoris. Angina indicates that the heart muscle isn't getting enough oxygen because of decreased blood flow. Angina is typically a heavy, oppressive sensation in the center of your chest. The discomfort can radiate to your lower jaw, one or both arms (usually the left), and the upper back and neck. Angina generally strikes during physical exertion or emotional stress and can last as long as half an hour. More typically, the discomfort subsides within a few minutes when the exertion or stress ends.

Angina may be a precursor of a heart attack, which occurs when prolonged oxygen deprivation leads to the death of a portion of heart muscle. The pain of a heart attack resembles angina but typically lasts longer and is a more severe, crushing sensation. A heart attack is often accompanied by clammy skin, sweating, nausea, shortness of breath, and weakness.

If you've never had chest pain before and it strikes during exertion, call your physician immediately. If symptoms don't subside with rest, head for the nearest emergency room. When a heart attack is coming on, every minute counts. Immediate treatment in the hospital can sometimes restore the flow of blood to the heart before serious damage occurs.

Finding the Cause

Because chest pain doesn't always come from the heart, it's crucial for physician and patient together to sort out the characteristics of the pain. What does the pain feel like? When does it occur? What makes it better? What makes it worse? What you tell your physician helps determine the diagnostic or therapeutic route to follow and may spare you needless and possibly harmful tests.

Children's Health

Constipated Child

Q. *For the past six months, our three-year-old son has averaged five days or more between bowel movements. We've tried to give him lots of natural fiber and fluids. On the advice of our pediatrician, we gave our son a stool softener for three weeks, but it hasn't helped. Should we keep using it?*

A. Prolonged use of a stool softener in children is not a good idea. Constipation in a three-year-old is a common problem. In addition to lack of fiber or fluid in the diet, possible causes include resistance to toilet training, painful anal fissures, or even Hirschsprung's disease (a lack of muscle tone in part of the colon). Ask your pediatrician to refer you to a pediatric gastroenterologist, who may be better able to diagnose and treat the problem.

Bed-wetting

Q. *My 11-year-old daughter occasionally wets her bed. Why is this happening, and what can we do about it?*

A. In most cases, the cause of bed-wetting is unknown. However, psychological stress from such changes as the birth of a sibling or separation from a parent is often responsible. That's especially likely if the child has begun to wet the bed again a year or more after being successfully toilet trained. Rarely, bed-wetting is caused by an underlying disorder, such as diabetes, infection, or seizures.

Once a physical problem has been ruled out, handle bed-wetting with gentle measures. Avoid mechanical devices that use frightening alarms and electric shocks. Limit fluids after supper. Be sure your daughter urinates just before bedtime. Wake her up to urinate several hours after she's gone to sleep. Praise and reward her for a dry night; don't scold or punish for a wet night. If the problem persists, a brief course of the drug imipramine (*Tofranil*) can help a child gain control by helping to close the urethral sphincter, the muscle that stops the flow of urine. Even if all those measures fail, most children outgrow bed-wetting by adolescence.

Cholesterol

Raising Low HDL Cholesterol

Q. *My "good" cholesterol (HDL) is usually below 35 mg/dl. I'd like to raise it to a healthier level, but I don't want to take drugs to do it. Is there some diet that would boost my HDL level without also raising my total cholesterol?*

A. No. Those foods that tend to increase HDL levels do the same for total cholesterol. But drug therapy isn't a particularly effective way to boost HDL, either. While some of the medications that lower total cholesterol may also raise HDL, that increase is generally slight, and no drug has yet been approved for that purpose. Moderate alcohol consumption—a drink or two a day—can raise HDL somewhat, but the drawbacks of taking up drinking outweigh that particular benefit. The best way to raise HDL is to exercise regularly; if you're overweight, lose weight; and if you smoke, stop.

Beta Blockers and Cholesterol

Q. *In a recent report on blood-pressure drugs, you discuss the effect of thiazide diuretics on blood cholesterol. What about beta blockers? I take*

Lopressor *to control hypertension, and I'm concerned because I have a very high cholesterol level.*

A. While beta blockers, including metoprolol (*Lopressor*), have been reported to raise triglycerides and lower levels of HDL (high-density lipoprotein)—the "good" cholesterol—it is unclear how great the effects are and how they might affect the prognosis for coronary heart disease. These changes do not appear to affect total cholesterol or LDL (low-density lipoprotein)—"bad" cholesterol—levels.

Cholesterol and Coffee

Q. *I've read that unfiltered brewed coffee can raise blood-cholesterol levels. But what about instant coffee? Can it raise cholesterol too?*

A. Probably not—although the evidence is scanty. The few studies that have focused on instant coffee found no link with cholesterol levels. But if you really want to be sure, you could pour your coffee through a filter before you drink it.

... and Tea

Q. *Is there any evidence on whether drinking tea affects cholesterol levels?*

A. While there have been no clinical trials to prove the point, several population studies suggest that tea does not raise cholesterol and may even lower it.

Cholesterol-lowering Drugs and Cataracts

Q. *My doctor wants to put me on medication to lower my cholesterol. But I read somewhere that the current cholesterol-lowering drugs can cause cataracts. Is that true?*

A. Only one cholesterol-lowering drug, lovastatin (*Mevacor*), has been associated with any risk of cataracts. And while that risk was believed to be quite low, the FDA advised users of the drug to get an annual examination for cataracts.

Yet several new studies have disproved any such association. The latest, a two-year study, found no difference between lovastatin and a placebo in forming cataracts. The annual examination for cataracts is no longer recommended for lovastatin users.

Cholesterol in Cheese . . .

Q. *What kinds of cheeses, if any, are acceptable for people trying to avoid too much cholesterol in the diet?*

A. There's not much cholesterol in cheese: An ounce typically contains about 20 to 30 milligrams. But cheese does have lots of fat: Most kinds get two-thirds or more of their calories from fat. (Low-fat cottage cheese is a big exception, with only 13 percent of calories from fat.)

So, if you're concerned about your blood-cholesterol levels, bear in mind that dietary fat is a much more important influence than dietary cholesterol.

There are some new, relatively low fat cheeses, but not all the ones labeled "light" really are. When checking a wide selection of cheeses, *Consumer Reports* found an enormous range in fat—from 0 to 83 percent of total calories from fat. To determine that percentage yourself, multiply the grams of fat by 9, then divide by total calories.

. . . and in Shellfish

Q. *Is it true that shrimp are high in cholesterol? What about other shellfish?*

A. A 3-ounce serving of boiled shrimp contains about 166 milligrams of cholesterol. (For comparison, one egg contains about 213 milligrams.) That's much higher than other types of shellfish, which range from about 60 to 90 milligrams of cholesterol.

On the bright side, however, shrimp weigh in at only 10 percent of calories from fat. And other shellfish are comparably svelte, ranging from about 5 percent of calories from fat for steamed lobster (without the butter dip, of course) to 16 percent for blue crab.

So, again: The amount of fat in the diet is much more important in regulating blood-cholesterol levels than the amount of total dietary cholesterol.

Cholesterol Levels and Ratios

Q. *According to my latest blood test, my total cholesterol level is 225 and my HDL level is 32. That's a ratio of 7:1. I've heard that a ratio higher than 4:1 indicates high risk. Should I be worried?*

A. Yes, but not about the ratio. It's the levels themselves that count: A total cholesterol level of between 200 and 240 puts you at moderate risk of coronary heart disease. And an HDL ("good" cholesterol) level below 35 compounds that risk. Some people can boost their HDL level by exercising, losing weight, and stopping smoking.

Confusion over HDL and LDL

Q. *You seem to discuss HDL and LDL as if they were two types of cholesterol. But then you say that both HDL and LDL transport cholesterol. I'm confused.*

A. The terminology is confusing. HDL (high-density lipoprotein) and LDL (low-density lipoprotein) are not types of cholesterol. Rather, they're fat-protein compounds that transport cholesterol through the blood. (HDL tends to carry cholesterol away from the arteries, thus earning the title of "good" cholesterol; LDL, or "bad" cholesterol, tends to deposit cholesterol in the walls of arteries.)

When cholesterol is attached to a lipoprotein, the entire complex is properly referred to as HDL or LDL cholesterol. Sometimes, though, HDL and LDL are used as shorthand terms to refer to the lipoproteins together with their cholesterol cargo.

Crystalline Niacin

Q. *You stated that "niacin—in crystalline or slow-release form— should be taken only under the careful supervision of a physician." My pharmacist has never heard of crystalline niacin. What is it?*

A. Crystalline niacin is simply "regular," short-acting niacin, also called nicotinic acid.

Eating Before Cholesterol Tests

Q. *I had my cholesterol tested recently at a health fair. The previous day, I ate two meals with lots of fat and cholesterol. Did that throw off my cholesterol reading?*

A. No. Total cholesterol levels don't change much from day to day. So you don't have to fast or worry about what you eat the day before a test. But if you were having blood drawn for a complete lipid analysis, including HDL cholesterol and triglycerides, then a 12- to 14-hour fast would be required.

Fish Oil for Triglycerides

Q. *In discussing fish oil for your heart, you indicate that "moderate" doses of fish oil can reduce triglyceride levels in the blood. What do you mean by "moderate"?*

A. "Moderate" means a daily dose of 3 to 10 grams of omega-3 fatty acids—the amount contained in about 6 to 30 fish-oil capsules. But such a dose could have the undesirable effect of increasing blood levels of LDL ("bad") cholesterol and could have other undesirable effects, such as decreasing the ability of the blood to clot. Moreover, the capsules could cost you from $500 to $2,500 a year. As we said, you'll be better off getting your fish oil by eating fish.

The Gallbladder and Cholesterol

Q. *My blood-cholesterol levels are high despite a low-fat diet. Could that have anything to do with the removal of my gallbladder 20 years ago?*

A. No. The gallbladder stores, concentrates, and regulates the flow of bile, which helps digest fats. But removing it has no noticeable effect on digestion and no effect at all on blood-cholesterol levels.

HDL from Food

Q. *We're constantly hearing about the opposing effects of high-density and low-density lipoprotein cholesterol in our blood, but when food is discussed, the distinction is dropped. Does the amount of HDL or LDL cholesterol in food affect the levels in our blood?*

A. No. Those lipoprotein-cholesterol combinations are broken down and reassembled within your body from their separate components—amino acids, cholesterol, and fats.

High Cholesterol, High HDL

Q. *I'm a 64-year-old man with a total cholesterol level of 225, despite a very low fat diet. My HDL and triglyceride levels are both 67. Since my HDL level is high, my doctor says I don't need to take cholesterol-lowering drugs. Do you agree?*

A. Yes. Based on the numbers you provide, your level of LDL cholesterol (the "bad" kind) would be about 145, which is only mildly elevated and not in need of reduction by medication. And since your level of HDL cholesterol (the "good" kind) is so high (normal for men is 35 to 45), your risk of coronary heart disease due to cholesterol is relatively low.

High Cholesterol, Low Risk

Q. *Last year, a lipoprotein analysis showed I had a total cholesterol level of 276 mg/dl, LDL of 188 mg/dl, and HDL of 77 mg/dl. My doctor says these results indicate a low risk of coronary heart disease. I eat a low-fat diet, I'm active, and my weight is good. Yet you have suggested that with such a high LDL level, drug therapy may be necessary for me. Is it?*

A. Probably not. As we said, before putting you on medication your physician should consider a number of variables, including your personal and family medical histories and any other risk factors for coronary disease. Based on your high level of HDL ("good" cholesterol) and your health habits, it sounds as if your risk factors are indeed well under control.

High-Cholesterol X Ray

Q. *I recently went to a chiropractor for lower-back pain. After taking an X ray, he asked me if I had a high cholesterol level. (At the time, I did have a total cholesterol reading of 246 mg/dl.) He pointed out some white spots along my spine and claimed they were plaque buildup in the blood vessels. Is that really possible?*

A. Yes. X rays can detect calcium in various organs and tissues, including the larger blood vessels. Your chiropractor probably saw calcium deposits in the wall of the abdominal aorta, the largest artery in the body. That could be caused by high cholesterol, aging, or both.

How to Lower Cholesterol

Q. *I have been taking Questran for several years. While this drug and a careful diet have helped to lower my cholesterol, it is still above 200 mg/dl. Recently I read an article that indicated one might lower cholesterol more effectively by taking Mevacor in combination with Questran. What do you think?*

A. Combination therapy of the kind you describe can be useful if one medication has proved only partially successful. Since cholestyramine (*Questran*) works in the intestinal tract and lovastatin (*Mevacor*) in the liver, combining them may make sense. Unfortunately, such combination therapy has not been studied as extensively as single-drug treatment. Each of these drugs also has side effects: Cholestyramine can cause constipation and bloating, while lovastatin can cause abnormal liver function and, less commonly, severe muscle aches. So regular monitoring by your physician should accompany such combination therapy.

Jumping Cholesterol

Q. *According to a finger-prick test, my blood-cholesterol level was 197. Two months later, it was 272 on a fasting blood workup. My diet didn't change during that time. Is such a jump possible in only two months?*

A. No. Cholesterol readings cannot vary that much, that soon. The finger-prick test was probably wrong. Squeezing the fingertip to draw blood produces secretions that dilute the blood and can lead to a falsely low reading.

Keeping Cholesterol Low

Q. *My husband has been taking Questran for a long time to lower his cholesterol, which is now normal. How long must he stay on this medication? It's quite expensive.*

A. Like most cholesterol-lowering drugs, cholestyramine (*Questran*) is effective only as long as it's used. If your husband stops taking it, his blood cholesterol would most likely return to its previous level—assuming all else stays the same.

Unfortunately, lower-priced generic versions of this drug are not yet available. Colestipol (*Colestid*) is another drug used to lower cholesterol; it *may* be cheaper.

Monitoring *Mevacor*

Q. *Five months ago, my doctor prescribed* Mevacor *to lower my blood cholesterol. Though I'm still on the drug, my doctor hasn't taken any more blood tests. Shouldn't they be done regularly to make sure the drug isn't affecting my liver?*

A. Yes. You need blood tests to confirm that the drug is keeping your cholesterol down and isn't impairing liver function. An interval of three or four months between tests is reasonable. Significant changes in liver function would require stopping the drug.

Niacin Alert

Q. *I recently read that the sustained-release form of niacin, which I've been taking to control my blood cholesterol, can cause liver damage. Why is this form of niacin dangerous, but the crystalline form, which causes me to flush, is not?*

A. It's long been known that both crystalline (short-acting) and sustained-release niacin can damage the liver at high doses. Evidence is now accumulating that the sustained-release form can cause liver injury even at low therapeutic doses. In several recent case reports, people who had recovered from such damage were then given crystalline niacin, with no ill effects. The reason for the difference is unclear; it may be that taking short-acting crystalline niacin allows the liver to recover between dosages while slow-release niacin affects liver enzyme systems for longer durations and with fewer recovery periods.

Another recent report suggests that high doses of niacin can aggravate diabetes and may induce the disease in borderline diabetics. Although niacin is available without a prescription, it should be taken only in crystalline form and under a doctor's supervision. Increasing the dosage very slowly to the target level will minimize uncomfortable facial flushing.

Psyllium to Lower Cholesterol

Q. *My friend takes a tablespoon of psyllium each day. He claims it lowers his blood cholesterol level. Is that really true?*

A. That has not been proved. Psyllium, a seed rich in soluble fiber, is the active ingredient in bulk laxatives such as *Fiberall* and *Metamucil*. The manufacturers have tried but so far failed to convince the FDA that ingesting psyllium is a safe and effective way to lower blood cholesterol. Until they do, they're not allowed to make any cholesterol-lowering claims.

Side Effects of *Lopid*

Q. *For two years, I've taken Lopid, which has lowered my cholesterol level from 280 to 230. My doctor wants me to keep taking it indefinitely. What are the long-term side effects?*

A. Gallstones, but they're rare. Even short-term side effects of gemfibrozil (*Lopid*) develop only infrequently; these can include digestive disturbances, impaired liver function, and muscle pains. If the drug hasn't caused side effects after two years, it probably never will.

Keep in mind, too, that if you decide to stop taking the drug, your cholesterol will probably shoot back up again.

Soaring Cholesterol

Q. *My 57-year-old wife has a cholesterol level of 520 mg/dl. We eat the same foods, and my blood cholesterol is only 170 mg/dl. Her blood pressure is normal, she's not overweight, and she doesn't smoke, drink, or have diabetes. After four weeks on* Mevacor, *her cholesterol level dropped to 340 mg/dl. But she developed painfully swollen ankles and now refuses to take this or any other cholesterol-lowering drug. What do you recommend?*

A. Swollen ankles are not a known side effect of lovastatin (*Mevacor*). Your wife should get back on cholesterol-lowering medication and look for another possible cause of her swollen ankles.

A blood-cholesterol level of 520 mg/dl is uncommon and ominous. Such high cholesterol, usually an inherited disorder, often causes coronary heart disease at a relatively early age.

Virtue by the Pint

Q. *I've been an occasional blood donor for several years. If I donate regularly, can I gain health benefits such as a lower blood-cholesterol level?*

A. Be satisfied with the intangible rewards. When it comes to donating blood, the health benefits accrue mainly to the recipient. As a donor, your body rapidly replaces the blood cells and fluid (plasma) you lose when you donate blood. The negligible amount of cholesterol lost along with the plasma is faithfully restored as well. The few people who may benefit from frequent bleeding have an uncommon blood disorder called polycythemia vera, characterized by an abnormally high red-blood-cell count. Periodic removal of blood is often a regular part of their treatment.

Zestril and Triglycerides

Q. *I'm a 54-year-old male and until recently had a triglyceride level of about 150 mg/dl, the high end of normal. Six months ago I started* *taking Zestril for high blood pressure. When last measured about a month ago, my triglyceride level was 427 mg/dl. Could Zestril have caused the increase?*

A. Probably not. Lisinopril (*Zestril*) is one of a class of antihypertensive drugs called ACE inhibitors, which are not known to affect triglycerides. Your elevated triglyceride level could arise from any of several factors, such as laboratory error, a failure to fast for 12 to 14 hours before taking the test, or weight gain.

Triglycerides and Diet

Q. *What type of diet will lower triglyceride levels?*

A. The same low-fat diet that can lower blood-cholesterol levels often lowers triglyceride levels as well. Avoiding alcohol and, for some people, cutting back on carbohydrates can also reduce triglyceride levels.

... and Estrogen

Q. *I'm a 65-year-old woman. My gynecologist wants me to take estrogen because the hormone would improve my cholesterol levels. But my internist warns that it would raise my triglyceride levels. What's the net effect?*

A. Overall, hormone replacement therapy helps protect women against heart disease. That's apparently because estrogen tends to decrease LDL, the "bad" cholesterol, and increase HDL, the "good" kind. It's possible that estrogen use might be even more protective if it didn't also raise triglycerides in some women. But for most women, the hormone's positive effect on cholesterol outweighs its negative effect on triglyceride levels.

Colon and Rectal Complaints

Colorectal Cancer Screening

Q. Recently, you said there's no evidence that screening tests reduce the death rate from colorectal cancer. But you also said they're still the best way to detect the cancer when it may be curable. I'm confused. Please explain the apparent contradiction.

A. It is clear that detecting a colorectal tumor early roughly doubles the chance of surviving for at least five years after surgery— from 40 percent to 80 percent, according to some estimates. And screening by sigmoidoscopy is the only way to find such tumors at an early stage. Until recently, no large, long-term studies have been published to prove that widespread screening reduces the overall death rate from colorectal cancer. Now, a new study of 1,100 patients—about a quarter of whom died of colorectal cancer—has provided the strongest evidence yet of the effectiveness of sigmoidoscopy. Published in the *New England Journal of Medicine*, the study found that patients undergoing at least one sigmoidoscopy test in the previous 10 years had a 60 percent lower risk of death from colorectal cancer than those who didn't have the test.

Anal Itching

Q. I have been suffering from severe pruritus ani for nearly a year. To find relief from the itching, I've been to a family physician, a proctologist, four dermatologists, and an allergist. So far, no treatment has helped. Do you know of anything that might relieve my discomfort?

A. Since you've already seen seven doctors, they've probably ruled out the most common causes of anal itching: worms, hemorrhoids, fungal infections, skin fissures, sweating, irritants in food, and poor anal hygiene.

One possibility that's sometimes overlooked is neurodermatitis. This is not an actual nerve disorder but rather a lengthy cycle of itching and repeated scratching. It leads to gradual thickening of the skin around the anus, which then itches more than ever.

If neurodermatitis is indeed the cause of your condition, it may gradually abate if you force yourself not to scratch the thickened skin. When you're at home, applying an ice-cold compress to the irritated area can ease the urge to scratch. Since many sufferers scratch when they're asleep, you should keep your fingernails short and even wear soft mittens to bed. If all else fails, a few sessions with a hypnotist or a psychotherapist might help you stop scratching.

Anal Fissures

Q. *I've been taking a tablespoon of mineral oil every night for many years to prevent anal fissures. Is this bad for me?*

A. Yes. Mineral oil decreases absorption of the fat-soluble vitamins (A, D, E, and K), and it can cause an unusual type of pneumonia if inhaled. Try a stool softener (*Dialose, Pro-Cal-Sof*) or psyllium laxative (*Fiberall, Metamucil*), which will minimize trauma to the anal area during bowel movements. Soaking in a warm bath for 10 to 15 minutes after bowel movements may bring some relief as well. Fissures that persist may require surgery.

Blood in the Stool

Q. *Microscopic traces of blood have been detected in my stool. Sigmoidoscopy revealed internal hemorrhoids near the entrance of the anus. Does this mean surgery, even though I've had no discomfort?*

A. Not necessarily. Stool softeners (*Dialose, Pro-Cal-Sof*) or psyllium laxatives (*Fiberall, Metamucil*) can reduce straining during bowel movements and may help stop the bleeding, just as they help prevent anal fissures. Antihemorrhoidal creams and suppositories are not particularly helpful for this problem. Like persistent fissures, persistent bleeding may require surgery.

Colonoscopy Pain

Q. *Because of a strong family history of colon cancer, doctors have advised me to have an annual colonoscopy. I've undergone the procedure a few times and found the pain nearly unbearable. My gastroenterologist says he doesn't give painkillers for colonoscopy. Is there anything that would help me cope with this ordeal?*

A. Yes—drugs, including those painkillers. Without them, the colonoscope causes discomfort and sometimes pain as it snakes through and stretches your colon. Before the procedure, most gastroenterologists give intravenous narcotics to kill pain and tranquilizers to relax the colon. If you can't persuade your gastro-enterologist to administer such medications, try another gastroen-terologist.

Diet and Diverticulosis

Q. *Like many people my age (over 50), I have diverticulosis. My doctor has told me not to eat seeds and nuts and to avoid constipation. But I know people with the same problem who have been told to eat, avoid, or do different things. Could you provide some insight into this problem?*

A. Diverticulosis is a common condition in which the inner lining of the intestine protrudes through the intestinal wall, forming small sacs or pouches in the colon. It affects one in four people by the age of 50 and is near-universal by the age of 80. It's believed that our modern low-fiber diet is at least partly to blame.

Diverticulosis usually doesn't cause any symptoms, but some people with the condition do experience bloating, cramps, and changed bowel habits, such as constipation, diarrhea, or alternating attacks of both. Abdominal pain (especially low on the left side) accompanied by fever might signal the development of diverticulitis, an infection of the sacs. That can lead to abscess formation and to perforation of the bowel, which can cause peritonitis, a generalized infection of the abdominal lining.

To avoid these problems, switch gradually to a higher-fiber diet that includes more whole grains, fruits, and vegetables. But omit the seeds and nuts your doctor mentioned; small and hard to digest, they can get trapped in the tiny pouches and cause inflammation.

Intestinal Bleeding

Q. *I have angiodysplasia of the colon. Can anything other than bran, psyllium* (Metamucil) *or olsalazine* (Dipentum) *help stop the bleeding?*

A. The recurrent bleeding that often follows angiodysplasia (swollen, deformed blood vessels in the intestines) can be stopped— but not by eating any foods or taking drugs, including the ones you mention. The only effective method is to cauterize the vessels with an instrument snaked up into the colon. While inserting the instrument may cause discomfort or pain, the cauterization itself is painless.

Ulcerative Colitis

Q. *I recently found out I have ulcerative colitis. What's the latest on the cause and treatment of this disease?*

A. Physicians still don't know what causes ulcerative colitis, an inflammatory disease of the colon that leads to diarrhea and rectal bleeding. (It can also affect the skin, eyes, and liver.) However, various drugs can suppress the inflammation and control the symptoms. These medications include the aspirinlike drugs mesalamine

(*Asacol*) and sulfasalazine (*Azulfidine*), corticosteroid drugs such as prednisone (*Deltasone*), and in resistant cases, immunosuppressant drugs such as mercaptopurine (*Purinethol*).

People who have had extensive ulcerative colitis for a long time may be at increased risk of colon cancer. These people should undergo periodic colonoscopy (inspection of the entire colon through a flexible lighted tube) to check for cancer or precancerous changes.

Cysts, Lumps, and Tumors

Benign Changes in the Breast

Q. *Six months ago I had a breast biopsy that showed benign changes—fibrocystic disease and intraductal hyperplasia. Is either of these linked to an increased risk of breast cancer in the absence of a family history?*

A. Your risk of breast cancer is no greater than average. The conditions you mention are natural changes that occur over time. Fibrocystic "disease," a term that indicates an abnormality or disorder, is a misnomer, since about half of all premenopausal women have it. It's really a catchall term for painful, lumpy breasts. Such lumps were once thought to be associated with increased cancer risk, but several studies have since dispelled that notion. Intraductal hyperplasia is a benign overgrowth of cells in the breast ducts, the tubes that carry milk to the nipple. Only when those cells start to appear abnormal on a biopsy does the risk of cancer increase.

Breast Lumps

Q. *At the time of my last routine physical, my doctor diagnosed a fibrocystic lump in my breast. I was told to avoid anything containing caffeine, including chocolate. But I love chocolate. Would eating chocolate really affect the growth of any lumps?*

A. Probably not. The theory that caffeine causes noncancerous breast lumps has never been proved. Besides, chocolate contains relatively small amounts of caffeine.

Fibroid Tumors and Estrogen

Q. *For years my doctor told me that I could never go on estrogen replacement therapy because I have a fibroid tumor on my uterus (roughly the size of a 14-week fetus). I've just reached menopause, and now he's changed his mind; he wants me to start hormone therapy. He says it would be okay—that the tumor would even shrink. Please advise.*

A. Estrogen can stimulate the growth of uterine fibroids, which are benign tumors of muscle and connective tissue that originate within the uterine wall. Now that you have reached menopause, your body's own supply of the hormone has begun to dwindle. Ordinarily, that would make the tumor shrink. The tumor might continue to shrink even with estrogen replacement therapy, if the dose of estrogen was relatively low. Higher doses might maintain the tumor or even make it grow.

If you decide to go on estrogen replacement therapy—because of severe menopausal symptoms, for example, or a high risk of osteoporosis or coronary heart disease—your fibroid tumor should be monitored closely. If it continues to grow, your physician may reduce your estrogen dosage or suggest that you stop taking the hormone entirely.

Body Bumps

Q. *I have several egg-shaped growths on my body. Please explain whether these bumps, diagnosed as lipomas, are dangerous and how the condition can be treated. I would have quite a few scars if the lumps were all surgically removed.*

A. Lipomas are benign, fatty tumors that are fairly common, typically appearing on the trunk, neck, and forearms. Usually they cause no discomfort and are best left alone. If you prefer to have them removed for cosmetic reasons, you can choose either conventional surgery or liposuction, in which a small tube inserted under the skin sucks out the fatty tissue, resulting in less scar formation. The rare lipoma that enlarges rapidly may harbor a cancerous growth, known as a liposarcoma, and should be removed surgically.

Dental Care

Dilute *Listerine?*

Q. *I have gum problems, so I use Listerine to control plaque. You reported a study suggesting that regular use of a mouthwash such as Listerine, which contains more than 25 percent alcohol, might increase the risk of oral and throat cancer. Should I dilute the stuff to neutralize that possible risk?*

A. Based on available evidence, we don't think that's warranted, especially for someone with gum disease. No one knows for sure whether the diluted formula would still fight plaque. All of the studies that established the effectiveness of *Listerine* for that purpose used it full strength.

Besides, as we pointed out, it's not clear whether there really is any cancer risk. That study from the National Cancer Institute was not conclusive. It compared 850 patients who had oral or throat cancer with more than 1,200 similar people who didn't. People who had habitually used mouthwashes containing more than 25 percent alcohol—the only ones are *Listerine* and its store-brand competitors—had a significantly higher risk for these cancers. But retrospective studies like this one can't prove a causal connection, and earlier, smaller studies of the same kind produced mixed results. An FDA panel is now reviewing the evidence.

Meanwhile, the most important risk factors for developing oral and throat cancer are still smoking, chewing tobacco, and excessive consumption of alcoholic beverages.

Alternatives to Tooth Caps

Q. *I have a gap between my two front teeth. Dentists have previously advised against grinding down two or four otherwise healthy teeth to cap them. Can anything else be done?*

A. There are new procedures for improving the appearance of your teeth without cutting them down or covering them with caps. Teeth can be reshaped, and spaces closed, by bonding with composites, porcelain, or plastic veneers. Ask your dentist about the relative cost and durability of the various procedures.

Braces: Health or Beauty?

Q. *Most children in my son's class have braces on their teeth, and our orthodontist is suggesting we have our son fitted, too. Are there good medical and dental reasons for giving children perfectly straight teeth, or is the main motivation cosmetic?*

A. It's mostly cosmetic. Crooked teeth can certainly cause emotional distress, particularly in appearance-conscious teens. But the reasons usually given for straightening a child's teeth—to prevent cavities and gum disease—have been questioned after a number of studies failed to show a protective effect. Nor have researchers convincingly linked crooked teeth to temporomandibular joint (TMJ) syndrome. Only a severely disordered bite is likely to cause such physical problems as difficulty chewing or gum disease.

Calcium for Oral Health?

Q. *I'm a 36-year-old woman with receding gums and bone loss around my teeth. My dentist recommends that I take calcium supplements to delay further bone loss. Is this the best treatment for my condition?*

A. There's no evidence that getting extra calcium will help reduce periodontal disease, which is what causes such bone loss. You should be evaluated by a periodontist. Treatment options range from periodic root planing to various surgical therapies.

Can Receding Gums Be Rebuilt?

Q. *I am almost 60 years old and have near-perfect teeth. But my gums are receding. I recall reading about an innovative technique in which a gumlike substance is attached to the teeth along the receding gum line. Can you tell me more about this approach?*

A. The technique you read about may have been guided tissue regeneration. A porous membrane placed between the gum and tooth encourages connective tissue to cross the membrane and bind to the root. The technique helps close periodontal pockets, the spaces between gums and roots where infection breeds. But such a procedure doesn't grow new gum tissue to cover the exposed roots. Currently, it can be used only in a few special cases.

Clean Teeth, Sore Mouth

Q. *Should my teeth and gums hurt after a cleaning appointment? Mine did for two or three days. My children had the same experience and didn't want to go back. We had this problem with a former dentist.*

A. In adults, a thorough cleaning may cause soreness that lasts a day or so. Some adults simply have sensitive teeth. Or, if periodontal disease exists, the dentist or hygienist may need to scale teeth well below the gum line, which can be temporarily irritating to the gums. Children, however, shouldn't have soreness after a cleaning.

Dental Planing vs. Cleaning

Q. *For some years I've had my teeth cleaned twice a year, at a cost of $25 to $35 per visit. A new dentist recently recommended that I have dental planing done. But the cost for planing is $120 a visit, and each visit deals with only one-quarter of my teeth. Please comment.*

A. There's a big difference between cleaning and planing, in function as well as cost. Cleaning removes tartar above and around the gum line and polishes the teeth. It's often performed by a dental hygienist. Planing, on the other hand, may be necessary to prevent the progression of gum disease. The procedure removes hard and soft deposits on root surfaces beneath the gum line and smooths, or planes, root surfaces. It's often performed under local anesthesia or nitrous oxide, and only by a dentist. For that reason, it costs much more than ordinary cleaning.

Dental X Rays

Q. *How often should I have dental X rays? My dentist says every six months is safe, but that strikes me as excessive—and expensive.*

A. If you're prone to tooth decay, you might need bitewing X rays as often as every six months. However, most people with healthy teeth can go one or two years between such X rays. Full-mouth X rays are generally needed much less often—about once every five years—to assess the overall health of the teeth and supporting tissue in adults. Modern X-ray equipment, as well as a lead apron and collar shield, minimizes the radiation exposure.

Fillings and Pins

Q. *When filling cavities in my teeth, my dentist installed pins to hold the fillings in place. Is this a new procedure, and is it really helpful?*

A. That practice has been around for quite some time. It's helpful when you've lost a good part of the tooth structure. The dentist threads pins into the tooth's dentin (the layer under the enamel) to serve as a support for the filling.

Fluoride for Toddlers: How Safe?

Q. *Until now I have used a damp cloth to wipe my 14-month-old daughter's teeth, but I'd like to start using a brush. The only kids' toothpaste I've found has sodium saccharin or fluoride in it. I'm afraid to use fluoride toothpaste before my baby can rinse out her mouth, since I read that swallowing fluoride toothpaste regularly can cause bone cancer over the years. And I'm not sure what sodium saccharin means. Can you please clarify?*

A. If used properly, fluoride toothpaste is perfectly safe for children. Over half the children in the United States already get fluoride in drinking water and, to a limited extent, in foods. They can theoretically get excess fluoride by swallowing toothpaste, but the only significant concern is the possibility of developing mild dental fluorosis—a harmless, whitish spotting of the teeth that occurs with excess fluoride intake over a period of years. A recent report from the Department of Health and Human Services found no convinc-

ing evidence that fluoride causes osteogenic sarcoma, or bone cancer. Still, there's no reason to put more toothpaste on the brush
than a child needs; use a pea-size dab (just enough to spread a thin
layer on the brush), then wipe it off with gauze.

As for sodium saccharin, that's just the familiar sweetener, saccharin, a common ingredient in diet products. In the tiny amounts
found in toothpaste, saccharin should be of no concern.

Fluoride Supplements

Q. *Are sodium fluoride supplements safe for my two-year-old child?*

A. Yes, in the correct dosage. Fluoride supplements (drops or
tablets) may be prescribed for children when the fluoride content of
local drinking water is less than 0.3 parts per million. The recommended daily dosage is 0.25 milligram up to the age of two, 0.5
milligram from age two to three, and 1 milligram from age three to
age 14, when the second molars have usually erupted fully. After
that, fluoride from toothpaste and fluoride treatments at the dentist's
office provide sufficient protection.

Some years ago, when the recommended dosage for children up
to age two was higher (0.5 milligram), there was some concern about
mild dental fluorosis—faint white spots on the teeth. But that minor
side effect rarely occurs today.

Implant or Bridge?

Q. *I have a lower molar that needs to be replaced soon. My dentist
has suggested a bridge, and said that bridges have been proved to be reliable. I'm interested in a more modern technique—getting a false tooth
supported by a pole implanted in the jawbone. How much research has
been done on this?*

A. Implants have an advantage over bridges, in that they don't
damage adjacent teeth. To install a bridge, the dentist must first file
down the adjacent teeth and then crown them. Single-tooth

implants have most often been used to replace upper front teeth, a procedure that is usually successful. However, the value of implants in replacing single back teeth has been less thoroughly studied. An implant can be used only if there is enough bone left under the gum to anchor it, and only in locations where the implanting procedure could not damage a nerve or sinus cavity. A dentist performing implants should have gone through a formal educational program in implant techniques.

The cost of implants and bridges is roughly comparable—generally around $3,000 for a single-tooth implant and a few hundred dollars less for a bridge. But some insurers that cover bridges do not cover implants.

Periodontal Surgery

Q. *My periodontist wants to trim back the gums around six of my teeth, although he says it's a gamble whether that will stabilize my periodontal disease. Friends have told me to save my money ($600 to $700) because it didn't work for them. Should I have the surgery?*

A. You can't predict the outcome of gum surgery from your friends' experiences. But you should consider surgery only after other measures have failed to stop the progression of the disease. Those measures include a combination of instructed self-care (brushing, flossing, dental rinse) and professional scaling and root planing. It would be wise to get a second opinion before you decide on surgery.

Root Planing

Q. *My dentist recently suggested I undergo root planing to cure gum disease. Is it really helpful or just a money-making gimmick?*

A. If there's a periodontal pocket—a space between tooth and gum caused by gum disease—root planing should indeed be helpful. The procedure removes any tenacious deposits of plaque and tartar below the gum line and scrapes away the infected outer layer of the root.

Saccharin Smile

Q. *After years of being told to avoid saccharin, I see it's in many toothpastes. Is it safe?*

A. Yes. The amount you'd ingest from toothpaste is insignificant.

Soda and Tooth Decay

Q. *A friend of mine says soda and other beverages that contain lots of sugar don't cause tooth decay. Is she right?*

A. Not quite. Sugary beverages are less damaging than sticky confections and even sticky fruits, particularly dried fruits. But soda contains acids that can erode the teeth. Drinking soda through a straw can help keep it off your teeth.

Sugar and Tooth Decay

Q. *In your report on sugar substitutes, you indicated that artificial sweeteners are not especially valuable in preventing tooth decay. Isn't too much sugar an important cause of tooth decay?*

A. Yes. Table sugar (sucrose), sugars in general, and indeed all fermentable carbohydrates can initiate dental decay. But because fluoride (in water, toothpastes, and rinses), plastic sealants for children, and improved oral hygiene have dramatically reduced the incidence of dental decay, sugar substitutes are now less important for preventing decay. It's still a good idea to limit between-meal intake of sugars, though, especially in sticky foods. The longer food particles stay in contact with your teeth, the more they promote dental decay.

Tartar Control

Q. *My dental hygienist told me that I have an unusually heavy buildup of tartar. Since I already floss nightly, she suggested that I try either an antiseptic mouthwash such as* Listerine *or a toothpaste containing baking soda, or else start flossing twice a day. What should I do?*

A. There's no need to floss twice a day, but be sure to use the proper technique when you do floss: Don't just work the thread between teeth with a sawing motion; curve it around each tooth and sweep it up and down across the broad surfaces.

Since you seem to develop tartar especially quickly, try brushing twice a day with a tartar-control toothpaste. (If you develop a rash around the outside of your mouth, try switching brands.) You might also use an antitartar rinse, such as *Colgate Tartar Control Mouthwash*, before you brush. Because these products contain chemicals that interfere with mineral crystallization, they slow the calcification of plaque into tartar by 30 to 40 percent. You should also continue to get periodic professional cleanings.

Listerine can fight plaque, but it doesn't slow the conversion of plaque to tartar. Toothpastes containing baking soda, or bicarbonate, may actually encourage tartar formation at least theoretically by increasing the alkalinity of the mouth.

Time for a Crown?

Q. *At my last checkup, my dentist told me that large silver fillings in two molars were deteriorating and that crowns would be necessary. Couldn't I just have the fillings replaced?*

A. Possibly, but that may not be the best solution. The average filling starts deteriorating after about 10 years. When you need a replacement, the tooth must be hollowed out further to accommodate the new filling. But if the old filling is large to begin with, removing more of the tooth could make it vulnerable to fracture from chewing. Often, the wiser choice may be a crown, which is more expensive than a filling but lasts much longer. The tooth is first filed down, and a crown made of porcelain, gold, or plastic is then anchored to the stub.

Toothpicks and Gum Disease

Q. *I thought brushing and flossing were enough to prevent gingivitis. But my dentist says I should also use a toothpick. Is that necessary?*

A. Brushing and flossing are usually enough for most people. However, a pick can help if your gums are still inflamed or if they bleed during cleanings, both signs of early gum disease. You can use a regular toothpick or a commercial "interdental stimulator," such as *Pick-A-Dent* or *Stim-U-Dent*.

Once a day, massage your gums by moving the pick in and out of the spaces between your teeth several times. Your gums may bleed at first, but after a few days the swollen tissues repair themselves to a healthier condition. If bleeding persists, see your dentist.

Tooth-Decay Defense

Q. *My children, ages 14 and 15, have no dental problems, but were recently advised by a new dentist to have their molars and premolars treated with sealants. What are the appropriate indications for this procedure?*

A. Sealants are an excellent way to protect children's first and second permanent molars, even in the absence of current dental problems. The procedure involves applying a soft plastic to the tooth surface to fill in the pits and fissures. This prevents food and bacteria from accumulating in those spaces. The plastic is then hardened with a special light or chemical.

Sealants should be applied soon after the molars appear: at about age six to seven for the first molar, and age 12 to 14 for the second. Children with evidence of tooth decay may also benefit from sealants on their premolars, also called bicuspids, which appear at age 9 to 12.

Wisdom-Tooth Removal

Q. *After a series of X rays, my dentist recommended removing my 13-year-old son's upper wisdom teeth at 15 for proper spacing. How seriously should I take this advice?*

A. This advice stems from the concern that impacted wisdom teeth, or third molars, will tend to push other teeth inward. But long-term studies have now shown that teeth can crowd together whether or not the wisdom teeth have been removed. Crowding, when it occurs, seems to result from a natural tendency of the teeth to move forward, although the exact causes are not clear.

Wisdom teeth should be removed when there is a better reason to do so, such as a painful infection around the teeth. Teeth that are merely impacted will not necessarily become troublesome over time. In addition, teeth that appear to be impacted at age 15 may right themselves in another five or six years. Since wisdom teeth generally don't reach their final position until the early twenties, it's too early to tell how your son's teeth will grow in.

⬜ OFFICE VISIT

Bad Breath: What Your Best Friend Can't Tell You

While performing a routine physical exam, I was having trouble checking the eyes of a new patient, a 42-year-old woman. She kept turning her head away. When I asked her to hold still, she stopped moving but took a deep breath and held it.

I stepped back and asked, "Are you worried about your breath?" Flushing, she nodded. I told her I smelled nothing offensive. She seemed relieved.

Bombarded by ads implying that people are secretly repulsed by our breath, most of us probably wonder whether we "offend." Such worry is usually needless. Halitosis, or true bad breath, is not a Madison Avenue myth, but it's much less common than the ads suggest. Few people have chronic halitosis, which is almost always caused by a dental or medical problem.

Natural Breath Odors

As I explained to my self-conscious patient, certain breath odors are common, but they're generally mild or temporary. If your breath is usually a little acrid or sour, for example, you've got plenty of company: From adolescence on, everyone's breath grows increasingly pungent.

Food can also taint your breath. What smells good on your plate may not smell good on your breath—even after you've brushed your teeth. Garlic or onion, the two main offenders, can stay on your breath up to 24 hours. That's because the active chemical in these foods travels through the digestive system to the blood, the lungs, and back out through the mouth. Even when rubbed on the skin, garlic will eventually find its way to the breath.

Sometimes, food particles can be the culprit. When particles of meat or other protein foods get stuck between the teeth, the particles eventually begin to rot. If brushing doesn't dislodge them, flossing will.

Smoking and drinking, of course, also leave their mark on the breath. But whether tobacco or whiskey breath is more offensive than, say, mint breath lies in the nose of the smeller.

If eating and drinking too much of some things are bad for your breath, eating too little is no better: Dieters may develop the mildly unpleasant "hunger breath" when certain metabolic waste products reach the lungs. (A snack curbs hunger breath but at some cost to the diet, of course.)

Then there's morning breath. While you sleep, your tongue moves less and saliva secretion slows almost to a standstill. Dead cells that line your mouth are no longer rubbed off, washed away, and swallowed. Bacteria break down those dead cells, releasing malodorous compounds. But the odor disappears as soon as you brush your teeth or have something to eat or drink.

A Whiff of Gum Disease

Dental problems are the most common cause of true halitosis. According to Consumers Union's dental consultant, Dr. Irwin Mandel, here is the typical odor-causing problem as well as a few ways to combat it:

If the mouth is not cleaned regularly, dental plaque—a sticky film composed mainly of bacteria—coats the teeth and can spread under the gum line. This can eventually create pockets between the gums and teeth where bacteria can break down protein and dead cells, causing offensive odors. Decaying blood from bleeding gums may intensify the odor.

If gum disease is threatening your teeth and fouling your breath, you'll need professional care. To help prevent such disease, keep your mouth clean. Here's how:

- ☐ Have your teeth cleaned professionally twice a year.
- ☐ Twice a day, brush along the gum line with a soft toothbrush angled 45 degrees toward the gums.
- ☐ Floss at least once a day.
- ☐ If these steps are inadequate, add a potent mouthwash. Thus far, studies have shown that two mouthwashes—*Listerine* and a prescription product, *Peridex*—significantly reduce the bacteria that cause plaque and bad breath. The effectiveness of other mouthwashes has not been established. Mouth drops and sprays can temporarily mask the odor—but might delay diagnosis of the underlying problem.

Dr. Mandel adds one last point about oral hygiene: The bacteria on your tongue don't contribute to gum disease, but they can cause bad breath. So if you're concerned about halitosis, gently brush the tongue, particularly if it's coated.

If Not Dental, Maybe Medical

If the dentist finds nothing wrong in your mouth, you may be one of the few people whose halitosis actually signals a medical problem. Most often, it's a local infection in your respiratory tract (the nose, throat, windpipe, and lungs), such as chronic sinusitis with postnasal drip or chronic bronchitis. Gastrointestinal problems, such as a hiatal hernia or a diverticulum (outpouching) of the esophagus, are occasional culprits.

Halitosis can also be caused by anything that dries the mouth—dehydration, fever, medications, salivary gland disorders, and even breathing through the mouth.

But don't let all this give you the wrong impression. Bad breath requiring the attention of a dentist or physician is uncommon. If you see your dentist regularly, your breath is probably nothing to worry about. Still, if you're worried as my new patient was, asking a professional might ease your mind. Your best friend may not tell you, but your dentist or doctor will.

☐ OFFICE VISIT
with Irwin D. Mandel, D.D.S.

Examining Your Dentist—and Finding a New One

The only thing worse than not seeing a dentist at all is seeing a bad one. Either way, you stand to lose your teeth. And if you stick with an inferior dentist, you'll lose your money as well.

Yet many people stay put when they should walk. Most of them probably don't even realize they're being inadequately treated, since that's not always obvious. To evaluate the kind of care you're getting, you'll have to ask yourself some probing questions. See if your dentist passes this dental exam:

Drilling and Filling

☐ *Is your dentist a talented technician?* Patients can't judge a dentist's technical skills precisely. But you can usually distinguish good dentistry from bad.

During prolonged probing or drilling, a good dentist will occasionally pause so you can relax and rest your jaw. After any sort of dental work, your bite should feel natural and your gums should not bleed. Fillings shouldn't catch your tongue, interfere with flossing, or give food particles and plaque a toehold.

If the dentist does the job well, a silver filling should last at least 10 years, depending on its size and location; crowns and bridges generally last even longer.

☐ *Does your dentist minimize temporary measures?* Be wary if your dentist puts in one temporary filling after another instead of proceeding directly to a permanent filling. This may mean the dentist has a high-volume practice and isn't willing to spend enough time with you. Or it may simply mean more visits, and thus more money.

Treatment and Overtreatment

☐ *Does your dentist discuss options?* Alternative treatments are more common in dentistry than in medicine. For example, a dentist may treat a tooth that has an especially deep cavity by doing root-canal work and then installing a silver filling; by inserting a gold inlay; by constructing a post and crown; or even by extracting the tooth. A good dentist should recommend the minimum treatment required to maintain dental health. When there are reasonable alternatives, your dentist should explain the pros and cons and let you decide.

☐ *Does your dentist respect your limits?* Tolerance for pain differs from person to person. If you can't bear the pain of dental work, your dentist should be willing to give you an adequate anesthetic or a sedative.

☐ *Does your dentist estimate and itemize?* Don't hesitate to ask for a written estimate of how long a proposed treatment will take and how much it will cost. After treatment, you should get an itemized bill.

☐ *Does your dentist avoid unnecessary work?* Certain shady practices can alert you to an overzealous dentist. Take your business elsewhere if your dentist:

1. Suggests replacing any silver amalgam fillings to protect you from the minute amount of mercury vapors they release when you chew. Overwhelming evidence supports the safety of amalgam fillings.

2. Wants to cut down several teeth and install crowns. (While that can be necessary in extreme cases, you should at least get a second opinion.)

3. Worries you about your appearance in order to sell you on some cosmetic dental procedure. (I'm all for cosmetic dentistry, but only if the motivation comes from the patient, not from the dentist.)

Preventing Trouble

☐ *Is your dentist prevention-minded?* This preventive approach should be apparent from the very first visit, when the dentist takes a thorough medical and dental history. Your dentist should also perform a complete "head and neck" examination at the initial visit and every few years thereafter. Such an exam should include inspection of your teeth, gums, jaw joint, facial muscles, and the inside of your mouth.

☐ *Does your dentist make you a partner in prevention?* Either the dentist or the dental hygienist should instruct you on how to care for your teeth. He or she should give you a refresher course from time to time, perhaps having you demonstrate your brushing and flossing techniques and suggesting improvements.

The dentist or hygienist should also advise you on such preventive extras as fluoride use, antibacterial rinses, and any supplemental oral hygiene aids you may need: an irrigator, a power brush, or floss threaders to clean around dental work.

☐ *Does your dentist invite you back?* A well-functioning recall system guarantees that no problem will go too far awry. In most cases, a checkup should be scheduled every six months to a year. At that time, the hygienist scales hardened plaque off your teeth and then polishes them. Unless something seems wrong, your dentist may not need to do much more than see that the hygienist has done a good job.

☐ *Does your dentist order X rays responsibly?* With most patients, there's no reason to take a full series of X rays more often than once every five years or so. A survey of decay with two to four X rays, called bitewings, may be taken every year or two, depending on your susceptibility to decay. If a problem arises, of course, X rays of the suspect area can be taken as needed. A dentist who never X-rays your teeth is just as bad as one who does it too often.

☐ *Does your dentist guard against infection?* Your dentist and hygienist should wear rubber gloves and a mask when treating you. Beyond that, your dentist should be willing to explain the other sanitation procedures used to protect patients and staff from infectious diseases.

How to Find a New Dentist

If your dentist fails your examination—or if you're moving or you don't have a regular dentist—you'll need to find a new one. Don't turn to the Yellow Pages or local dental societies; they list dentists but don't evaluate them. Instead, try these sources:

☐ If there's a dental school nearby, call and ask for the names of practicing faculty members.

☐ If a hospital or health center provides dental services in your area, ask the dentist in charge for recommendations.

☐ If you already know an orthodontist or periodontist, ask for the name of a good general practitioner. Those dental specialists should be familiar with the quality of work done by referring dentists.

☐ If you're moving and your current dentist meets most of the criteria I've discussed, ask whether he or she can recommend colleagues in your new location.

When you visit a dental office for the first time, the dentist and staff should be willing to answer all of your questions. If they're not, that's one sign that you ought to look elsewhere.

☐ Diabetes

Diabetes and Blood Sugar

Q. I'm a 42-year-old man, and my fasting blood sugar level is about 115–125 mg/dl. I have no family history of diabetes, am not overweight, and have had normal results on glucose-tolerance tests. But I'm afraid I may develop diabetes if my blood-sugar level stays high. How can I lower it?

A. Other than stopping any medications (such as corticosteroids or thiazide diuretics) that might be boosting your blood sugar, there's really no way to lower your sugar level. But there's also no reason for you to try. Your fasting blood-sugar level is barely elevated: A normal level can range up to 120 mg/dl; the threshold for diagnosing diabetes is 140. All you need is to keep doing what you're doing— and get tested once a year.

Diabetic Neuropathy

Q. I have diabetes, which has caused excruciatingly painful neuropathy. Apart from painkillers, can anything help?

A. Unfortunately not. Many supposed cures—including a variety of vitamins—have been tried, but there's no evidence that any of them works.

The accumulation of sorbitol in nerve fibers is probably what causes diabetic neuropathy (diseased nerves). In people without diabetes, only a small amount of glucose in the blood is converted to sorbitol, a more complex sugar. But since people with diabetes don't use glucose normally, more of it gets changed to sorbitol. Experimental trials using drugs that block the conversion of glucose to sorbitol have been disappointing thus far, but newer versions of those drugs may yet prove helpful.

Diet and Nutrition

Too Much Iron?

Q. *I have been warned against taking iron-containing vitamin and mineral supplements. Supposedly, men and postmenopausal women cannot excrete the iron, and excessive levels of the metal accumulate in their blood. Is this a real concern?*

A. Not if you take your iron as part of an ordinary vitamin pill. The amount of iron in most multivitamin or multimineral supplements is relatively small—usually 18 to 27 milligrams, or 100 to 150 percent of the U.S. recommended daily allowance (RDA) for adults. However, the amount of iron in pills "with iron" is 10 to 15 times the U.S. RDA. That large a dose, commonly used to treat people with anemia, could lead to serious iron overload in a person without a medical need for extra iron. Increased iron stores may be a coronary risk factor in men.

While a little supplemental iron won't hurt you, you probably don't need it. Most Americans get enough of the mineral from red meats, chicken, beans, sardines, and iron-fortified breads, cereals, and flour.

Too Much Liver

Q. *Because I have trouble tolerating supplemental iron tablets and injections, I've thought of adding large portions of liver to my diet instead. Is this safe, or do I risk ingesting harmful amounts of chemicals and hormones?*

A. While liver is nutritious, a steady diet of it can be hazardous. The primary risk isn't from any exotic chemical or hormone but from too much vitamin A. A 6-to-9-ounce serving of beef liver supplying the recommended daily allowance (RDA) for iron also packs some 18,000 to 27,000 micrograms of vitamin A. That's up to 34 times the normal RDA for the vitamin. This much vitamin A daily would lead to toxic levels in the body over time. The same portion of liver also contains roughly 800 to 1,200 milligrams of cholesterol. That's equivalent to the amount in four to six eggs—more than double the average daily intake of cholesterol and far above amounts permitted in cholesterol-lowering diets.

Apart from any risk, it's unlikely that you'd be able to eat enough liver to correct a significant iron deficiency. For example, the minimum therapeutic dose of iron prescribed for iron-deficiency anemia is typically about 130 milligrams daily—nearly nine times the RDA for women.

No Meat with Potatoes?

Q. *I've heard that you shouldn't combine foods that contain protein with foods that contain carbohydrates at one meal. Is there any sound basis for such advice?*

A. None whatsoever. After all, even individual foods are in themselves combinations of protein and carbohydrates, as well as fat.

Elevated Potassium

Q. *Blood tests show that my potassium levels are higher than the maximum normal level of 5.5 millimoles per liter. I follow good health habits, including a careful diet. What could be causing that elevation?*

A. By far the most common reason is simply a faulty testing technique that churns the blood while drawing or analyzing it. This in turn releases potassium from the blood cells. However, the elevation might also be caused by potassium supplements, medications (such as certain diuretics, beta blockers, or ACE inhibitors), kidney failure, insufficient secretion of adrenal hormones, or any one of several uncommon inherited diseases.

If repeated blood tests confirm that your potassium level is indeed above normal, you should be evaluated to find out what's wrong. Any further rise can be dangerous.

Frozen Bacteria

Q. *Does freezing destroy bacteria in food?*

A. No. Although growth stops and the total bacterial count may decline during freezing, plenty of microbes will survive. If frozen foods aren't safe before freezing, they won't be safe after thawing. Heat is the surest way to kill bacteria. The temperature and cooking time depend on the food.

Frozen Vegetables

Q. *You've reported that frozen vegetables are often more nutritious than the fresh ones sold in supermarkets. And you said not to thaw them before cooking, so they'll retain nutrients. But how can I be sure frozen vegetables haven't thawed and refrozen at some point before I buy them?*

A. Feel the bag to make sure the vegetables aren't clumped together. If the bag is clear, check to see that there's no sign of ice crystallization inside. Boxed vegetables, of course, are forced into clumps, so it's harder to tell if they've thawed and refrozen. All you can do is avoid boxes with lots of ice crystals on them.

Honey vs. Sugar

Q. *Is honey nutritionally superior to plain table sugar?*

A. Not at all. In fact, honey and table sugar are nearly indistinguishable chemically; once digested, they're identical. Neither sweetener has any nutritional value other than calories. Teaspoon for teaspoon, however, table sugar actually contains fewer calories than honey (16 vs. 22). That's because the dry crystals take up more space than the dissolved sugars of honey.

Lactose Intolerance

Q. *What diet should a person with lactose intolerance follow?*

A. Without the enzyme lactase, the body is unable to break down milk sugar (lactose) into simple sugars that can be absorbed. People deficient in this enzyme can't completely digest milk and milk products, especially cheese and ice cream. Small amounts of those foods usually cause no problem, but too much can result in cramps, bloating, diarrhea, and flatulence.

If you're highly intolerant to lactose, you can take lactase capsules or tablets (*Dairy Ease, Lactaid, Lactase*) before you ingest milk products. *Lactaid* is also available as a liquid concentrate that you add to regular milk. And lactose-reduced milk (also sold under the brand name *Lactaid*) is available in food stores.

Pick-Me-Up Pill

Q. *Five years ago I began taking one tablet of Vivarin each morning as a substitute for coffee. Occasionally I take another in the afternoon for a quick boost. Is this drug as safe as coffee, as the label claims?*

A. Yes—if you're not overly sensitive to caffeine. A *Vivarin* tablet contains 200 milligrams of caffeine, about the same as two cups of brewed coffee. In some people, though, even a single cup of brewed coffee can cause side effects such as nervousness, irritability, and rapid heartbeat.

Processed vs. Natural Sodium

Q. *In your article on nondrug therapies for hypertension, you suggest that people with high blood pressure avoid salty foods. You listed some foods that are surprisingly high in sodium—including celery. Doesn't the sodium in a natural food have less effect on blood pressure than the sodium found in processed foods?*

A. Sodium has the same effect on blood pressure, whether it's consumed as table salt, in processed foods, or as it occurs naturally in foods. Some researchers have suggested that there might be a difference, but the weight of the evidence suggests otherwise. If you're monitoring your sodium intake, add up sodium from all sources. Celery does have more sodium than most vegetables (about 35 milligrams per stalk), but that's still not a lot.

Raw Fish: Angling for Trouble

Q. *How great a risk is there, if any, in eating sushi and sashimi?*

A. Raw fish may be contaminated with potentially harmful bacteria or with parasites, which can cause even more serious problems. There's a small risk that raw fish dishes may contain parasitic worms, which can cause abdominal pain, impaired absorption of nutrients, and even anemia. Freezing the fish at minus 10°F for 72 hours destroys parasites, but home freezers may not sustain such a low temperature. For that reason, it's best not to prepare raw fish yourself. You can cut your risk by avoiding fish most likely to harbor parasites: carp, salmon, trout, cod, and Pacific rockfish.

Generally, it's safer to eat raw fish dishes at a restaurant. But there's no way to guarantee that the restaurant you choose—or its supplier—will have properly frozen and handled the fish destined for you.

Too Little Iodine?

Q. *Because I have a family history of hypertension, I do not cook with salt. Since most table salt is fortified with iodine, I am concerned that my family may not be getting enough iodine. Should we be concerned?*

A. No. The U.S. recommended daily allowance (RDA) for iodine is small and easily met even on a low-salt diet. Shellfish and saltwater fish, as well as breads (which are made with iodized salt), provide significant amounts of the mineral. You'll also obtain trace amounts from almost everything you eat, since fruits, vegetables, and plants used for livestock feed are often grown in areas where the soil is rich in iodine.

Too Much Tuna?

Q. *I have been eating 3½ ounces of tuna daily for at least a year. I recently read that tuna contains mercury and can be a health hazard if eaten more than five times a week. Is this true?*

A. Yes, but mainly for pregnant women. Considering the average level of mercury present in tuna, a safe limit would be about 3 ounces of tuna a day, or 20 ounces a week, according to guidelines established by the FDA. But that limit actually includes a large safety margin. It's calculated to protect the population most vulnerable to mercury toxicity: fetuses exposed through their mothers' diets. So your tuna intake alone isn't likely to cause problems. But if you also eat large amounts of other mercury-rich fish, such as swordfish and trout, you may want to have your blood-mercury level tested as a precaution. Excessive intake of mercury can cause insomnia, anxiety, and minor tremors. The FDA limits the amount of mercury permitted in commercially sold fish, but federal regulations don't apply to sport fish.

Too Much Vitamin D

Q. *I'm postmenopausal, and a bone-density scan has revealed moderate osteoporosis. I've been advised to take 100,000 I.U. of vitamin D every week and a combination of Premarin and Provera. I also take 1,500 milligrams of calcium a day. What are the risks of this regimen? Is it effective against osteoporosis?*

A. Except for the vitamin D, your regimen offers some benefits. *Premarin*, an estrogen product, is indeed effective in slowing osteoporosis. Taken by itself, however, it increases your risk of uterine cancer. *Provera*, a synthetic progesterone-like medication, helps protect against that complication. Taking extra calcium is also beneficial if you don't obtain about 1,000 milligrams daily in your ordinary diet.

However, such a megadose of vitamin D is unnecessary and can cause calcium to be deposited in your soft tissues; it can also put you at risk for kidney stones and kidney failure. Though vitamin D does enhance calcium absorption, you need only about 200 I.U. a day, especially since estrogen has a similar effect. Two glasses of milk a day, combined with ordinary exposure to sunlight, could easily meet your needs.

Too Much Zinc?

Q. *My ophthalmologist suggested taking zinc for age-related macular degeneration. I already take a multivitamin supplement that includes 50 milligrams of zinc. I also have a separate supply of 50-milligram zinc tablets. If I take both supplements, would the 100-milligram daily dose be excessive?*

A. It could be. Daily intake of zinc at levels only slightly higher than the U.S. recommended daily allowance (15 milligrams for men, 12 for women) may cause subtle adverse effects. In two studies, for example, as little as 18 to 25 milligrams of supplementary zinc a day reduced body levels of copper, an essential trace mineral. In another study, daily zinc supplements of 80 to 150 milligrams reduced HDL cholesterol, the "good" cholesterol that lowers the risk of coronary heart disease. Somewhat higher doses of zinc have produced immune-system impairment and other adverse effects. For those reasons, the Food and Nutrition Board of the National Research Council advises against taking daily zinc supplements above the RDA "without adequate medical supervision." Meanwhile, evidence of zinc's value for your eye problem remains unproven.

Vegetarians and Vitamins

Q. *I've recently decided to become a vegetarian. What vitamin supplements should I be taking?*

A. That depends on how strict a vegetarian you plan to be. If you eat eggs, dairy products, or tempeh (a fermented soybean product), there's no need for vitamin supplements. If not, you should take vitamin B_{12} tablets. The recommended daily allowance is 2 micrograms daily.

Vitamins Forever

Q. *For several years, I've been taking supplements that include high doses of the B vitamins and vitamin C. Since you've indicated that vitamin supplements are necessary only in a few special cases, I may stop taking them. But I've read elsewhere that doing so can create what amounts to a vitamin deficiency. Is that true?*

A. No. Taking vitamin supplements doesn't create increased demand. And any excess of the B vitamins and vitamin C are excreted in the urine. When you stop taking supplements, your body will simply get its ration of vitamins the natural way—from the foods you eat.

Warnings on Diet Drinks

Q. *Some diet sodas and juices contain the notice* "PHENYLKETON-URICS: CONTAINS PHENYLALANINE." *What is phenylalanine—and why the warning?*

A. Phenylalanine, which is an essential amino acid needed by the body, also happens to be a component of the sweetener aspartame. Most people needn't worry about the warning, but phenylalanine can be a problem for the one in 15,000 who suffer from a metabolic disorder called phenylketonuria (PKU). These people lack an enzyme needed to process the amino acid, which can reach toxic levels in their blood and tissues if dietary sources are not restricted. Accordingly, the FDA requires products with aspartame to bear a warning. Screening for PKU at birth is routine. Mental retardation can result if a newborn's PKU goes undiagnosed.

Why Not Canned Fruit?

Q. *Everything I read about proper diet calls for fresh fruit. What's wrong with canned fruit?*

A. Processing the fruit reduces the amount of certain vitamins somewhat, particularly vitamins A and C. And fruit that is canned without the skin has less fiber than fresh fruit. In addition, fruit is often canned in syrup, which adds calories. Still, canned fruit—especially when it's canned in its own juices—is a lot better than no fruit. Use it as a substitute for out-of-season fresh varieties.

How Much "Caf" in Decaf?

Q. *I've heard that decaffeinated coffee has as much as 30 percent of the caffeine in regular coffee. Is that true?*

A. No. The decaffeinating process actually leaves behind only about 3 percent of the caffeine. A cup of decaf has 2 to 5 milligrams of caffeine, compared with 40 to 108 milligrams for regular instant and 110 to 150 milligrams for drip-filtered. You'd have to drink an enormous amount of decaf to feel any effect from the caffeine.

The Color of Carrots

Q. *I eat a lot of vegetables, particularly carrots. Sometimes my skin gets a yellow tinge. I've been told that I should stop eating carrots when that starts to happen. Should I?*

A. Only if you don't like the color. While eating large quantities of foods that are high in beta carotene—especially carrots—can color your skin yellow, that doesn't indicate any kind of harmful reaction. And it's totally reversible. In fact, you don't have to stop eating these foods altogether to make the yellow discoloration disappear; just cut back a bit on carrots and take up the slack with other vegetables. After a few weeks, your skin should begin to clear.

Moldy Bread

Q. *If there's a spot of mold on a slice of bread, is it safe to break off that spot and eat the bread?*

A. No. With a soft food like bread, simply removing the visible mold won't necessarily remove all of the spores. If ingested, those mold spores might cause gastrointestinal problems, such as diarrhea.

However, you can safely excise a small moldy area from firm foods, such as hard cheese, salami, and some fruits and vegetables. Be sure to include at least a half-inch margin of safety all around.

Fat and Cholesterol in Foods

Q. *My nonfat yogurt lists 5 milligrams of cholesterol. How can a food have cholesterol but no fat?*

A. It's possible, but uncommon. Foods that have no fat—including most fruits, vegetables, and grains—generally don't contain cholesterol either. Nonfat yogurt and skim milk are among the few exceptions.

Many more foods, especially those that contain vegetable oils, have fat but no cholesterol. That's because cholesterol is found only in animal products such as meat, eggs, milk, and cheese. And that's why it's no trick for a bag of fatty potato chips or even a package of margarine to boast "no cholesterol."

Fat Beer?

Q. *Does beer contain any fat or cholesterol?*

A. No. The calories in beer (about 150 per 12-ounce can of regular beer and 100 for light beer) come from alcohol, carbohydrates, and a minuscule amount of protein.

High-Fat Infant Formula

Q. *I was astonished to see that coconut oil is a major ingredient in Enfamil and other top-selling infant formulas. Isn't this oil extremely harmful to the arteries? Why would anyone feed it to a baby?*

A. It's true that Americans have been advised to cut back on foods containing coconut oil and other highly saturated fats, which have long been linked to coronary heart disease. But at this time, these guidelines apply only to older children and adults. Babies under age two need fats to meet energy needs and to supply the raw material for cell membranes. Infant formulas contain 30 to 50 percent saturated fatty acids, about the same as breast milk.

Is Buttermilk Fatty?

Q. *How does buttermilk compare to plain milk in calories and fat content?*

A. Favorably. Commercial buttermilk is usually made by adding lactic acid to either low-fat or skim milk. (The acid sours and thickens the milk.) An 8-ounce glass of buttermilk made from low-fat milk contains about 2 grams of fat, which accounts for 18 percent of the 100 total calories; buttermilk made from skim milk usually contains less than one gram of fat, accounting for less than 9 percent of the 80 total calories, a negligible amount. By comparison, a glass of whole milk contains 8 grams of fat, or about half of its 150 calories.

Minimum Fat Intake?

Q. *We hear so much about the desirability of limiting fat intake to no more than 30 percent of calories consumed. But surely fat must play some vital role in the diet. Isn't there a minimum fat intake below which nutrition would suffer?*

A. Yes, but no one knows exactly what that minimum level is. Clearly, some fat in the diet is needed to build parts of the body's cells, particularly the cell membranes. In animals, diets with virtually no fat can retard growth and cause skin disorders. In certain cultures, however, people consume as little as 10 percent of total calories from fat with no apparent ill effects.

Mono- and Diglycerides

Q. *Many food products claim to be fat-free but list mono- and di-glycerides as ingredients. Aren't they fats?*

A. Yes. But they're added in tiny quantities, usually to keep baked goods soft. "Fat free" really means virtually fat-free—less than one gram (9 calories) of fat per serving, an inconsequential amount.

Calories in Low-Fat Yogurt

Q. *It seems odd that low-fat plain yogurt doesn't always have fewer calories than regular yogurt. Is that because of the milk solids added to low-fat yogurt?*

A. Yes. On average, yogurt made from low-fat milk has about 40 percent less fat than regular yogurt. But the added milk solids give it about 50 percent more protein and carbohydrates. That's why we reported five extra calories—145—in a cup of low-fat plain yogurt vs. 140 in a cup of regular yogurt. However, each of these amounts represents an average compiled by the U.S. Department of Agriculture. The actual number of calories in a serving of yogurt varies widely from brand to brand.

Eat More "Healthy" Fats?

Q. *I have a question regarding "healthy" fats. What are the best sources to ensure sufficient intake of essential fatty acids?*

A. Nutritionists have definitely identified two essential fatty acids—components of fat that cannot be manufactured by the body and thus must be obtained from food. These are linoleic and linolenic acid, found in seed and vegetable oils. Other possible essential fatty acids include arachidonic acid, which is found in meat, and eicosapentaenoic acid (EPA), found in fish and seafood.

Unless you've discovered a way to remove all the fat from your diet, you're probably getting more than enough of these nutrients already. Any attempt to increase your intake of fats, even "healthy" fats, is likely to do more harm than good.

Digestion and Indigestion

Eating Around Ulcers

Q. *I have a duodenal ulcer. What foods and beverages should I avoid?*

A. People who have a duodenal, or peptic, ulcer usually produce excessive secretions of gastric acid, especially at night. So anything that prompts the stomach to secrete even more acid is likely to be harmful and cause discomfort. The main dietary culprits include alcohol and beverages that contain caffeine, such as coffee, tea, and cola drinks. (Decaffeinated coffee also stimulates the production of gastric acid.)

Calcium-containing foods and beverages, including milk and milk products, initially neutralize gastric acid. But an hour or so later, there's often a rebound effect and acid secretion actually increases. (For that reason, you shouldn't take a calcium carbonate antacid such as *Tums* to ease an ulcer; you'd be better off with a noncalcium product such as *Riopan* or regular *Rolaids*.)

In addition to avoiding items that stimulate gastric acid production, another way to minimize acid secretion is to eat several small meals a day, rather than two or three large ones. Contrary to popular belief, while certain things you eat or drink can aggravate an ulcer, no food or beverage has been shown to *cause* ulcers.

Bile Without a Gallbladder

Q. *In a recent report on gallstones, you explained that the gallbladder stores bile produced by the liver and sends it into the small intestine to help digest fats. But you didn't explain where the bile goes when a person's gallbladder is removed. Can bile still aid in digestion—and can it form stones elsewhere?*

A. Yes and probably not, respectively. When the gallbladder is removed, bile will flow directly from the liver via the bile ducts into the small intestine, where it continues to aid digestion. Stones tend to form when chemically imbalanced bile is stagnant, as it is when stored in the gallbladder. They rarely form in the bile ducts, and never in the intestine.

Caffeine and Heartburn

Q. *After reading your recent pain reliever report, I found that my usual pain reliever, Excedrin II, contains 65 milligrams of caffeine. I've noted before that caffeine seems to aggravate my heartburn problem. What do you suggest?*

A. Cut down on caffeine—and cut out the *Excedrin*. Caffeine can stimulate the production of stomach acid, a common cause of heartburn. In your case, the best choice for an occasional pain reliever would be acetaminophen (*Anacin-3, Tylenol, Valadol*), since that drug is less likely than aspirin or ibuprofen to cause gastrointestinal symptoms. As we said in our report, the addition of caffeine has not been proved to make a pain reliever more effective.

Don't "Chooz" Antacid Gum

Q. *I've used Chooz antacid gum for years and wonder why you didn't mention it in your antacid report. Does Chooz have the same effects as other antacids containing calcium carbonate?*

A. Yes—and then some. In addition to its main ingredient, calcium carbonate, *Chooz* also contains peppermint oil. This substance may aggravate heartburn by relaxing the sphincter muscle between the stomach and the esophagus. We recommend you choose something else.

Flatulence

Q. *I've recently begun suffering from flatulence. I'm 65 and have no obvious digestive problems. What could be causing this often embarrassing problem?*

A. It could be the food you eat. Rectal gas is the price some people pay for good nutrition.

Intestinal bacteria can ferment the remnants of certain foods, thereby producing gas. Likely foods include bran and whole grains, as well as many fruits and vegetables, such as apples, avocados, beans, broccoli, cabbage, cauliflower, corn, cucumbers, melons, onions, peas, peppers, and radishes. Sometimes milk and other lactose-containing products (ice cream, puddings, custards) are at fault. Try cutting out suspect foods for a while, and see if it helps.

Swallowed air can also produce a small amount of gas. It may help to eat slowly, chew with your mouth closed, and avoid gulping food. Over-the-counter remedies such as simethicone (*Mylicon*) and charcoal tablets are of little help.

Flatulence is usually nothing to worry about unless it's accompanied by a recent change in bowel habits such as constipation or diarrhea. That could indicate an underlying disorder such as an intestinal infection or tumor, irritable bowel syndrome (spastic colon), or poor food absorption.

Herniated Esophagus

Q. *My husband has had a burning sensation in his throat. It was diagnosed as a herniated esophagus, but I didn't understand the doctor's explanation. What is it, and what can be done about it?*

A. Your husband is suffering from reflux esophagitis, or heartburn inflammation of the swallowing tube due to stomach acid coursing back up. Sometimes the problem is related to a hiatal hernia, in which the stomach protrudes through the diaphragm into the chest. It can also result when the sphincter muscle at the lower end of the esophagus doesn't close properly.

Your husband should avoid irritants, including alcohol, aspirin, citrus juice, and coffee (caffeinated and decaffeinated). He should also avoid fats and peppermint, which tend to relax the sphincter muscle. He can help to reduce abdominal pressure by losing weight or wearing loose-fitting clothes. And he should take advantage of gravity to keep stomach acid where it belongs: Elevate the head of the bed on 4-inch blocks, and don't lie down after meals.

Certain medications can help. These include antacids, such as *Maalox*, *Riopan*, and *WinGel*; acid-blocking drugs, such as cimetidine *(Tagamet)* and ranitidine *(Zantac)*; and drugs that strengthen the lower esophageal muscle, such as metoclopramide *(Reglan)*.

Rice and Bananas

Q. *I have irritable bowel syndrome. In your book* The New Medicine Show, *you refer to "the time-honored treatment of rice and banana" as a way to reduce the severity of diarrhea. What, exactly, is this treatment?*

A. It's a dietary regimen in which those two low-residue foods are eaten almost exclusively for a few days to ease a short-term bout of diarrhea. Diarrhea resulting from irritable bowel syndrome may also respond temporarily to this diet. (Paradoxically, the syndrome sometimes responds to a high-fiber diet as well.) However, since irritable bowel syndrome tends to recur, medicines to reduce intestinal spasms may be a better way of treating diarrhea caused by the ailment. Limited use of prescription drugs such as dicyclomine (*Bentyl*) and hyoscyamine sulfate (*Levsin*) can be helpful.

Sorbitol and Digestive Problems

Q. *I've heard that sorbitol can cause digestive problems. Is that true?*

A. Yes. Sorbitol, a mild natural sweetener used in gum, candy, and many foods, is absorbed slowly by your digestive system. Because it remains in the gastrointestinal tract for up to eight hours, it may be broken down by bacteria in the large intestine. If you consume lots of sorbitol, excessive gas and diarrhea can result.

Test for Liver Disease

Q. *For several years, blood tests have shown that I have a slightly elevated level of the liver enzyme known as SGPT. But all of the other tests for liver disease have found nothing wrong with me. My doctor says it's not uncommon for a healthy person to have an elevated SGPT count. Is he right?*

A. Yes. Usually there's no known cause. (In obese people, it may be due to accumulation of fat in the liver.) Assuming you've been tested for hepatitis, including the newer test for hepatitis C, you have nothing to worry about. However, your liver should be retested periodically to make sure it remains healthy.

Stomach-Acid Reflux

Q. *For many years I have suffered from indigestion. All tests have come back normal except one, a stomach X ray that demonstrated "min-*

imal reflux." My doctor suggested I wear loose-fitting clothes and eat smaller meals, but I still have the problem. Is there anything else I can do?

A. Reflux means the sphincter muscle separating your stomach and esophagus isn't closing properly, thus allowing stomach acid to course up into your esophagus. Symptoms include a sour taste in your mouth and heartburn. Your doctor's advice was designed to reduce the pressure on your abdomen. You may get additional relief by losing weight, sleeping with the head of your bed slightly elevated, and avoiding lying down right after meals.

If necessary, drugs might also be considered. Metoclopramide (*Reglan*) strengthens malfunctioning muscle. Cimetidine (*Tagamet*) and ranitidine (*Zantac*) decrease the production of stomach acid. Antacids can be used after meals and at bedtime to neutralize stomach acid.

🖸 OFFICE VISIT

When Your Belly Hurts

One evening, I received two phone calls within minutes of each other. Both callers were patients of mine, generally healthy men in their midforties. Both of them had diffuse belly pains, accompanied by nausea and repeated vomiting. And both had had an appendectomy in the past. There the similarity ended: The first man also had diarrhea and fever; the second didn't. Which one was sicker?

You might think the fellow with more symptoms was in worse shape. But this man's fever and diarrhea—two signs of probable infection—actually made me breathe easier. By the next morning, his symptoms were starting to subside. The problem appeared to be mild gastroenteritis—intestinal flu—that cleared up in a couple of days.

The other man was in real trouble. Shortly after we hung up, I met him in the emergency room. Examination and X rays indicated complete blockage of his small intestine. He was rushed to the operating room, where the cause of the blockage turned out to be a band of scar tissue from his previous appendix operation. The surgeon cut the band and relieved the obstruction. Another few hours, and that segment of the bowel might have died for lack of circulation.

Belly pain can be a confusing symptom. There are many organs in and around the abdomen, and any of those organs can hurt. You can't always judge the severity of the problem by how bad the pain is, how sick you feel, or how many other symptoms you have.

Still, there is information that can help you figure out whether you should call your doctor right away or try to treat the problem yourself for a while.

Probably Not Serious

The most common causes of abdominal pain are generally the least serious, even though they often produce disabling symptoms.

Intestinal flu, for example, can cause pain, nausea, fever, vomiting, and diarrhea. But the symptoms usually subside in two to three days. The most prevalent kind of food poisoning causes similar symptoms and runs an even shorter course, usually without fever. Both of those intestinal infections produce generalized belly pain rather than pain confined to one area. If the symptoms are tolerable and wane within a day or so, there's probably no need to call a doctor. You can relieve the pain with acetaminophen *(Tylenol)* and the diarrhea with loperamide *(Imodium)*.

Certain pain relievers, often used in high doses for arthritis, are another common cause of belly pain. Should you develop pain in the central part of your upper abdomen while you're using ibuprofen *(Advil, Nuprin)* or aspirin, stop taking it immediately. If the problem is just a mild stomach inflammation, the belly pain should disappear within a few days, with the help of an over-the-counter antacid. (However, ibuprofen or aspirin can also cause a serious problem— stomach bleeding. That shows up as blood in the stools, described below.)

Signs of Danger

One sign that you may need medical help is pain that's confined to one area of the belly. Such pain is more likely to involve a single organ than pain that's diffuse or that moves from area to area. And problems that involve a single organ are more likely to be serious.

Call your doctor immediately when abdominal pain is accompanied by:

Severe weakness, dizziness, and sweating. These are all signs of internal bleeding, either from the stomach or bowel or from a ruptured aorta.

Bloody stools. They might indicate an ulcer, blockage of a major blood vessel to the bowel, or telescoping of one segment of the bowel into another. Bleeding from the stomach usually results in black stools; rapid or lower-bowel bleeding will turn the stools reddish. (Iron supplements or *Pepto-Bismol* can also blacken the stools, whereas beets and cranberries can turn them red.)

Possible pregnancy. Pain could indicate a spontaneous abortion or an ectopic pregnancy (one that's developing outside the uterus).

A bulge in the wall of the groin. It could mean a strangulated hernia.

Chills and high fever. That could signal peritonitis, a severe infection of the entire abdominal lining caused by a ruptured appendix or diverticulum.

Bloody urine. That's a sign of kidney stones.

With or without these symptoms, sudden and severe belly pain that doesn't let up merits a doctor's attention. Even when belly pain is mild, you should still call your doctor if it persists for more than two or three days or recurs over a period of more than a week or two.

☐ OFFICE VISIT

Easing Irritable Bowel Syndrome

An aspiring young pop singer was telling me about a health problem that threatened her career, forcing her to miss rehearsals and even cancel a few performances.

Ever since she had returned from a gig aboard a Caribbean cruise ship six months before, she had been plagued by alternating bouts of diarrhea and constipation. She experienced abdominal pains before bowel movements, often felt bloated, and was embarrassed by gas. She thought she might have picked up some intestinal infection in the tropics.

But my patient also confided that she had had bowel problems before, especially at stressful times, such as during school exams or before an audition. A doctor once told her she had a "nervous stomach." She was afraid that I would label her a hypochondriac if I found nothing wrong with her physically.

I assured her that emotional factors could not be causing her symptoms, although stress or worrying about the problem could be making them worse. I'd check for parasites and other possible causes. But it sounded as if she had irritable bowel syndrome, a common disorder that afflicts as many as one in five adults in the United States.

Diagnosing the Syndrome

Doctors used to attribute irritable bowel syndrome to anxiety or depression. That was partly because people with the condition have no evidence of physical disease other than their intestinal symptoms and partly because anxious or depressed people are more likely to seek medical attention for those symptoms. Overall, however, there's no evidence that people with irritable bowel syndrome have more psychological problems than the average person. What actually causes the syndrome in the first place remains unknown.

Before I could diagnose irritable bowel syndrome in my patient, I first had to check for various underlying disorders involving the lower intestinal tract that can cause similar symptoms. Blood and stool tests ruled out any parasites or bacteria that she might have brought back from the tropics. A short trial on a restricted diet ruled out intolerance to lactose (the sugar in dairy products), which stems from a deficiency of *lactase* (the intestinal enzyme that breaks down the sugar). Careful questioning excluded a possible intestinal reaction to excessive amounts of sorbitol or fructose, often used as sweeteners in low-calorie products.

The other main possibilities were more serious: gynecological disorders, such as endometriosis; inflammatory bowel disease, such as ulcerative colitis or Crohn's disease; and even colon cancer. But her overall good health and normal blood tests suggested that she didn't have any of those disorders, so expensive testing was not warranted at that point.

I diagnosed her problem as irritable bowel syndrome and started treatment to relieve her symptoms.

Self-Help for Symptoms

Irritable bowel syndrome can cause three different types of problems: constipation, diarrhea, and a combination of abdominal pain, gas, and bloating. Some people with the syndrome experience only one symptom; others go back and forth from one to another. Still others have the pain-gas-bloating complex plus either diarrhea or constipation at different times. Fortunately, most people diagnosed with irritable bowel syndrome can treat themselves, depending on their symptoms:

☐ *Constipation* is the most common symptom of irritable bowel syndrome. Note that a daily bowel movement is not necessary for good health. If you aren't bloated and you move your bowels without discomfort, you're not constipated, no matter how infrequently you defecate.

When constipation is a problem, extra fiber in the diet usually helps. That's because fiber absorbs water and swells in the bowel, creating bulkier stools that stimulate bowel contractions. People who are constipated should gradually add fiber to their diet over several weeks until they're consuming about 20 to 30 grams a day. (If you're eating more fiber, you should probably drink more fluids, too.)

Good sources of fiber include wheat bran, whole grains, whole-grain breads, and certain fruits and vegetables, notably raspberries, pears, peas, and brussels sprouts. Prunes are especially effective bowel cleansers, since they're not only high in fiber but also contain an irritant that rouses the bowel muscles.

If dietary measures alone aren't sufficient, a bulk laxative containing psyllium *(Fiberall, Metamucil)* can sometimes help. But avoid regular use of other types of laxatives, such as saline products *(Citroma, Phillips' Milk of Magnesia)* or stool softeners *(Colace, Surfak)*. Over time, those laxatives can weaken bowel function. As a result, many people with chronic constipation become dependent on the drugs, which can have significant side effects ranging from potassium depletion to liver damage.

☐ *Diarrhea,* often containing mucus, is probably the easiest symptom to treat. Again, dietary modifications can help bring relief. In this case, however, you should cut back on fresh fruits and vegetables that contain lots of fiber and eat more complex carbohydrates, such as potatoes, pasta, and white rice. If dietary measures fail, a few doses of over-the-counter loperamide *(Imodium)* will usually do the trick. Again, don't rely on medication any longer than you have to. (See your physician if you notice blood in the stool; that can signal a more serious disorder.)

☐ *The pain-gas-bloating complex* is the most distressing manifestation of irritable bowel syndrome and the most difficult to treat. A bowel movement usually relieves the pain, but cramps often return soon after. People who suffer from this set of symptoms apparently have increased sensitivity to normal amounts of intestinal gas. Even small amounts of food produce abdominal distention, or bloating.

The first step in treating this complex is to try to identify and cut out any foods that might be causing gas. The most common offenders include beans, brussels sprouts, cabbage, and onions. But the culprits vary from person to person, and you might have to do some detective work yourself. Some physicians recommend simethicone *(Mylicon)* or charcoal tablets, but I've found that those drugs usually don't help.

Beyond Self-Help

If dietary measures and judicious use of nonprescription drugs don't bring relief, your physician can prescribe stronger drugs. For example, an antispasmodic medication may help people whose pain stems from intestinal spasms. But all you may really need from your doctor is reassurance that nothing is seriously wrong with you physiologically or psychologically. Irritable bowel syndrome almost always subsides on its own and often doesn't return for long stretches.

When I last saw my patient a few months ago, she had made several dietary changes and was coping with her problem successfully. She was less concerned about the symptoms that remained, and she had returned to the stage.

☐ OFFICE VISIT

Relieving Constipation—
If You Really Have It

On a summer night in 1937, the boys in bunk six were getting ready for bed. Our horseplay stopped abruptly when the camp nurse entered, clipboard and pencil in hand. Muffled giggles punctuated the silence as she interrogated each of us in turn. "Hard, medium, soft, or none?" she asked. She wasn't taking egg orders—she was checking our bowel movements. Anyone foolish enough to answer "hard" or "none" was rewarded with a dose of castor oil.

Although that barbaric ritual has gone the way of public hangings, the obsession with daily bowel movements and the rampant overuse of laxatives continue. Bombarded by ads linking empty bowels to a full life, Americans spend about $300 million a year on the more than 700 brands of over-the-counter laxatives. Much of that money is spent needlessly, because of tenacious misconceptions about constipation.

One myth is that waste products can contaminate the rest of the body if they're not eliminated frequently. More than 60 percent of Americans believe that a daily bowel movement is necessary for good health. Actually, the frequency of bowel movements among healthy people varies greatly—from three a day to three a week. If you aren't bloated and you move your bowels without discomfort, you're not constipated, no matter how infrequently you defecate.

Constipating Habits
When constipation does occur, it's more likely to strike older than younger people and women more often than men. In some cases,

it reflects an underlying medical problem: Constipation can be caused by hormonal disorders, such as an underactive thyroid gland; elevated blood levels of calcium; neurological injuries or disorders; or mechanical blockages of the bowel, such as hemorrhoids or tumors.

Usually, however, constipation is caused not by disease but by life-style and habits. The most common problem is too little fiber in the diet. Fiber absorbs water and swells in the bowel, creating bulkier stools, which stimulate the bowel contractions that push the stool along.

People who are constipated should consume about 20 to 30 grams of fiber a day. (If you're eating more fiber, you should probably drink more fluids, too.) Good sources of fiber include wheat bran, beans, whole grains, whole-grain breads, and certain fruits and vegetables. Prunes are not only high in fiber but also contain an irritant that rouses the bowel muscles. Eat them sparingly, or they can cause "rebound" constipation when you give them up.

Inactivity can also contribute to constipation. Exercises such as jogging, aerobics, and brisk walking are good ways to stimulate the bowel, but any increase in activity will help.

Bowel movements are not just something your body does; you have to pitch in, too, by heeding the urge to defecate. Rather than rushing to catch the train right after breakfast—when the urge to defecate is often strongest—try to set aside enough time to let nature take its course.

A host of common medications can be constipating. They range from iron or calcium supplements and aluminum antacids to prescription drugs, including antidepressants, antihistamines, antispasmodics, narcotics, tranquilizers, and heart drugs such as calcium channel blockers, diuretics, and antiarrhythmic agents. If you became constipated soon after you started taking medication, ask your doctor whether drugs could be the cause and what to do about it.

Constipating Laxatives

Although the cavalier use of castor oil has declined, the myth of the benign, "safe and gentle" laxative lives on. Used regularly, all methods of purging the bowel—enemas as well as laxatives—tend to weaken bowel function and cause dependence. Research suggests that about half the people who use laxatives regularly could regain normal bowel function by discontinuing those drugs. And all laxatives can have significant side effects. Laxatives should be avoided if possible or used only occasionally.

Temporary constipation may crop up when travel or illness disrupts your normal habits, when there's a change in your diet, or when you're taking a short course of medication. The problem often resolves itself in a few days. If not, an enema or laxative can help. In any case, your accustomed bowel movements will generally return when you resume your normal routine.

If you've been constipated for more than two or three weeks without apparent cause, consult your physician. After ruling out serious disorders, your doctor will help you design a program of dietary and other life-style changes. If that doesn't work, an enema or laxative may be required.

Doctors

D.O. vs. M.D.

Q. *What's the difference in training between an osteopath and a medical doctor?*

A. Doctors of osteopathy (D.O.'s) are similar to doctors of medicine (M.D.'s) in training, licensing, and scope of practice. The major difference between them is philosophical. Osteopathic physicians place greater emphasis on the role of the musculoskeletal system (bones, muscles, and tendons) in the healthy functioning of the human body. In addition to using conventional diagnostic and therapeutic procedures, they may use manipulation techniques to diagnose and treat medical problems.

☐ OFFICE VISIT

Second Opinions Make Good Medical Sense

The diagnosis was breast cancer, but the prognosis was good. The woman was past 60; she had reached an age when the mortality rate from breast cancer declines sharply. The tumor was relatively small, and no lymph nodes were felt in her underarms.

Her main concern was her appearance after surgery. Would she lose her breast?

Yes, said the surgeon who examined her. Because the tumor was located in the center of the breast, just behind the nipple, he explained, the best surgical course was a mastectomy, or breast removal.

Couldn't the tumor be removed without taking the entire breast?

In the surgeon's opinion, the odds against a good cosmetic result with a lumpectomy (removal of only the tumor plus a margin of normal breast tissue) in this case were too great. Besides, a lumpectomy would require a follow-up course of radiation therapy— something not usually needed after a mastectomy. Finally, he said, full breast removal would probably be needed in the end. He advised an immediate mastectomy rather than risk the need for additional surgery.

The Second Opinion

Unreconciled, the woman sought out the chief of surgery at a nearby medical center. He had a different view. "I almost never perform mastectomies anymore," he said. "In my experience, women do just as well with a more limited operation." He expressed confidence that the tumor could be successfully removed without a mastectomy. The chance of a recurrence, already small, would be reduced further by X-ray therapy after the operation. The woman opted for the lesser procedure, with good results.

Which surgeon was right? Probably both were. The advice given by doctors is not always based on scientific certainty about the best course of treatment. They sometimes base their advice on their own clinical experience and that of their colleagues—perhaps even on their confidence (or lack of confidence) in their ability to perform a procedure successfully. That's why second opinions make good sense whenever the patient feels uncertain about a recommended course of treatment.

When to Get One

Most second opinions on surgical procedures explore nonsurgical options or the surgical alternative that is best. I usually recommend a second surgical opinion for procedures about which professionals often disagree. These include surgery on the back, breast, ear, knee, nose, prostate, and veins, as well as coronary bypass and hysterectomy (with or without removal of the ovaries).

But it's important that you approach a second opinion with realistic expectations: Only occasionally will you find, as the breast-cancer patient did, a difference of opinion as well as an alternative that coincides with your own hopes.

Insurance companies sometimes require second opinions for certain surgical procedures in the hope of reducing unnecessary surgery and its costs. Yet they've found that savings rarely materialize. It turns out doctors actually agree on the course of treatment about 95 percent of the time.

Why this high rate of concurrence?

Insurers believe that doctors fear a disagreement might lead to a malpractice suit or to a loss of referrals. Doctors view the high rate of agreement as a sign of growing professional consensus on medical treatment. But it may also be that patients often seek second opinions about procedures that are clear-cut, where differences of medical opinion do not exist.

Even when there are no therapeutic alternatives to sort out, a second opinion can be of value. It can provide a fresh perspective if there's a vexing clinical problem. Or it can confirm a diagnosis or the wisdom of a course of treatment, and thus ease any doubts you—or your physician—may have.

So don't hesitate to tell a doctor you want another opinion. He or she should welcome it. If you sense reluctance or defensiveness, all the more reason to seek another opinion.

How to Get One

While friends and relatives may offer help, the best choices are likely to come from a primary-care physician who has your interests at heart. Ask that physician for the names of two or three experts in the field, preferably doctors who are affiliated with a university-connected medical center or a large, nonprofit community hospital outside your local area. Distance lends independence to a medical viewpoint.

If you don't have a personal physician, then call such a medical center or hospital on your own. Ask to speak to the chief of surgery, if you want an opinion about a surgical question, or to the chief of medicine, if your questions concern a nonsurgical course of treatment.

You can use the *Directory of Medical Specialists,* a publication available at most public libraries, to check the background and qualifications of any specialist to whom you are referred.

You can also get a referral from your county medical society or from a medical society outside your area. The latter source increases the chance that a second opinion will not be colored by some concern for the feelings or interests of the original physician.

Here are other sources:

☐ The federally sponsored Second Surgical Opinion Hotline (800-638-6833) has a national index of medical organizations that provide referrals on surgical questions.

☐ The Health Benefits Research Corporation also offers a Second Opinion Hotline (800-522-0036) as well as a referral service. A fee of $185 includes the cost of consultation with a board-certified specialist.

You must be able to talk freely with whoever gives you a second opinion. Explain what you've already learned, and provide him or her with the results of any tests. If the second opinion concurs with the first, you probably know enough to make your final decision.

More opinions won't make bad news any better.

When Opinions Differ

If opinions differ, don't rush to a third source—you're not taking a poll. Instead, ask the first two to support their opinions. You're looking for scientific evidence drawn from published clinical studies, not just personal anecdotes.

When the facts aren't clear—or when the two physicians interpret the same facts differently—going to a third source makes sense. Ask that third physician why the first two opinions differ—and for help in reaching your decision.

The Decision Is Yours

Armed with the facts, you may very well decide against elective surgery, or choose a nonsurgical alternative.

If the choice involves surgical procedures with similar success rates and all other factors are equal, let your physician's comfort level decide. There's no reason for you to help a surgeon sharpen new skills on an unfamiliar technique.

☐ OFFICE VISIT

Dialing Your Doctor

Early one morning, you phone your doctor. After a half hour of busy signals, a receptionist answers and, without asking whether your call is urgent, puts you on hold. Several minutes later, there's a click and a dial tone.

You call back and eventually reach an assistant who asks about your problem. He or she says the doctor is busy and will return your call at the end of the day. But the call never comes. When you try again, the office is closed. You finally hear from the doctor around noon the next day. After you hang up, you realize that you didn't have enough time to describe your symptoms adequately.

Sound familiar? My guess is that most patients have had similar frustrating experiences trying to get through to their physician over the phone.

Some of that frustration is inevitable. Surveys show that 10 to 15 percent of the contacts between patients and their physicians now takes place over the phone. One out of every three prescriptions for children and one out of every 10 for adults are now dispensed by telephone calls among patient, pharmacist, and physician.

Usually, people call their doctor because they're sick—sometimes too sick to come to the office, but more often not sick enough to need an office visit. Or they phone about side effects of medications or about medical news they've heard. They phone for a referral to a specialist or for laboratory test results. And they phone for opinions about friends or relatives who are ill.

A busy internist or family practitioner might receive 20 to 30 calls a day from patients. Since the average return call lasts nearly five minutes, a doctor can easily spend around two hours a day just calling patients back. On top of that, physicians get calls from other doctors, and some physicians initiate their own follow-up calls to patients.

Little wonder that the process sometimes gets fouled up, particularly if the office staff is inexperienced or the phone system itself is inadequate. If busy signals, crossed signals, and ignored messages become commonplace, it's time to protest or even switch doctors. But there are ways to minimize unanswered calls and to make the most of your time on the phone with your doctor.

Getting Through

Keep these points in mind when you have to reach your physician:

☐ *Emergencies.* Most physicians will accept your call if you say it's an emergency. Don't let the office staff dispute your need for rapid attention. Insist on speaking with the doctor immediately, and ask to stay on the line until the doctor picks up the phone.

Of course, in the case of a life-threatening emergency—a suspected heart attack, severe bleeding, or difficulty breathing—you should call an ambulance, not your physician.

☐ *Nonemergency calls.* Few physicians accept routine phone calls during busy office hours, since the interruptions make it difficult to care for patients in the office. Some physicians set aside special hours for taking calls from patients. But most doctors prefer to call you back, preferably at a specified time. You'll save yourself a lot of aggravation by asking your doctor ahead of time what's the best way to reach him or her by phone.

If the doctor can't speak with you immediately, leave your number and request a return call. Don't let the secretary tell you to call back later. When you do call back, all too often the doctor will have left for the day.

When you leave a message, don't accept "later" as an estimate of when the doctor will call back. Ask the secretary for an approximate time. If that time is inconvenient, tell the secretary when you can be reached—and keep your line open then. If the physician doesn't phone at the specified time, call the office again.

□ *After hours.* When the office is closed, you'll reach the answering service, and the covering physician will return your call. Covering doctors know that off-hour calls are often emergency calls, so they try to respond quickly. But if you don't hear from the doctor soon, don't hesitate to call the service again.

Say It Right

When you do get your physician on the phone, you'll probably have only a short time to get your point across. Here's how to use that time to your best advantage:

□ Think about what you want to say beforehand. Since you may receive the call at a time when your thoughts aren't well organized, consider jotting them down.

□ Keep your medication bottles near the phone so that you can read off the names and dosages of your prescriptions.

□ Know the phone number of your pharmacy in case your doctor wants to call in a prescription. And keep a pencil and paper near the phone for recording any medical advice you receive.

□ In describing your symptoms, stick to what you consider the most important ones. But describe those main symptoms precisely. Don't lead off with a minor complaint; describe the symptom you're most concerned about first. The unfortunate fact is that many doctors will place greatest importance on what you mention first.

☐ Get it all out. In one study of 74 visits to various physicians, researchers found that doctors interrupted more than two-thirds of the patients within 18 seconds. Over the phone, the urge to break in may be even stronger. Insist on having enough time to describe your problem without interruption.

☐ OFFICE VISIT

Speak Up to Your Doctor

Are you satisfied with your doctor? If so, you're like most people. One survey found that even though people complain about the health-care system in general, most are satisfied with their own physician. But the fact that you trust or feel comfortable with your doctor doesn't necessarily mean you're getting the best possible care.

A longtime patient of mine, a 48-year-old accountant, always insists that I take charge. I have to draw his symptoms out of him. Whenever I offer a choice of treatments, he smiles and says, "You're the doctor, you tell me." He generally seems quite satisfied with my care and has referred many patients to me over the years. On one recent visit, however, he seemed uncomfortable.

A month earlier, I had prescribed a diuretic to lower his elevated blood pressure. But the pressure stayed high. I asked him about his use of the medication. After several evasive answers, he blurted out that he'd stopped taking it because it made him tired. When I asked why he hadn't called me, he said he'd been reluctant to complain about a drug I'd recommended. He thought it might "hurt my feelings."

While it's important to be satisfied with your doctor, satisfaction does not guarantee good health. In fact, one study found that satisfied patients were less healthy than dissatisfied ones. And in my experience, satisfied patients are no more likely to comply—for example, to take their medications or stick with their special diet—than dissatisfied patients.

A Compliant Patient

But it's also not enough just to comply with your doctor's orders. Consider this case: A 53-year-old teacher was started on hormone therapy by her gynecologist to help prevent osteoporosis and heart disease. Shortly thereafter, she became nervous, irritable, and unable to sleep. The gynecologist, concerned that she might have an overactive thyroid, referred her to me.

Tests ruled out hyperthyroidism. Reassured that she had no serious disorder, the woman confided the source of her anxiety. A close friend had died recently of breast cancer. When the woman's gynecologist mentioned that hormone therapy might pose a small risk of the disease, she became frightened. But the gynecologist had made the therapy seem so important that she just took the pills and kept her fears to herself.

The woman's unquestioning compliance had not only kept her from discussing her fears but also from asking pointed questions about the treatment. Such questions might have led her gynecologist to reconsider the hormone prescription. Or they might have led the woman to seek a second opinion.

I suggested we measure her bone density and blood-cholesterol levels. The results, combined with her medical history, showed no need for hormone treatment, and it was terminated. I urged her to increase her calcium intake and to keep exercising.

The Active Patient

In both of these cases, the problem was a reluctance to speak up. In an elaborate series of recent studies, patients were taught to play a more active role with their doctor. The studies were the first experimental test of the idea that such active participation might actually improve patients' health.

Researchers from Boston's New England Medical Center pooled data from four separate trials involving a total of more than 250 patients who had either ulcers, high blood pressure, diabetes, or breast cancer. All of the patients were assigned to an experimental group or a control group. The breast-cancer patients were assigned according to when they showed up at the hospital; the others were assigned randomly.

In the experimental group, specially trained research assistants coached patients just before two separate office visits. To get patients involved in their own care, the assistants showed them the medical record of their previous office visit, identified issues that patients may not have understood the last time, and urged them to ask the doctor to explain.

The assistants described various treatment options and encouraged patients to inquire about those options during the visit and to negotiate the decision. They also emphasized that patients were free to bring up anything related to their problem, including its impact on their everyday activities or on their emotional, sexual, or family life. To help patients overcome their reluctance to speak out, the assistants had them rehearse their questions and negotiation strategies aloud.

In the control group, the assistants gave patients only general information about their disease.

Not surprisingly, patients who were urged to be more assertive obtained more information from their doctors. More important, the coached patients had significantly better outcomes. They reported fewer limitations in what they could do, and better overall health. They also did better on the two objective measures that were taken: The coached patients with hypertension had lower blood pressure than the controls, and those with diabetes had lower blood sugar.

Becoming an Active Patient

Active, outspoken patients, who ask for explanations, seek information, and aren't reluctant to get second opinions, are usually less afraid of their disease and more determined to fight it. And they do indeed seem to do better than their passive counterparts. Here are some ways to become a more active patient:

- ☐ Don't worry that asking questions or expressing your reservations about treatment will annoy or disappoint the physician. You've come to the office to care for your health, not to please your doctor. If the doctor refuses to address your questions or reservations, consider looking for another physician.
- ☐ Prepare for your office visit by writing down the key features of your problem and the questions you want to ask. If you tend

to feel shy or nervous with the doctor, rehearse the questions at home and then again in the waiting room.

□ Ask about the reasons for tests or X rays and about their meaning and accuracy; about the risks and benefits of treatment; and about the side effects of medications and their possible interactions with other drugs, or with food or drink. Be sure you understand everything the doctor says. If the terms are too technical, request a translation.

□ Ask for written information about your disorder. Or read about it at the library. Knowing about your problem will help you assert yourself in the doctor's office. And the more you know, the more intelligently you're apt to follow—or question—your doctor's advice.

☐ OFFICE VISIT

How to Talk to Your Doctor About Symptoms

The office visit is rarely a meeting of equals. You may have had to wait a week or more for the appointment. Uncomfortable, nervous, and worried, you sit in the waiting room with a crowd of unhappy strangers. Then you're led into an examining room, where you undress and wait some more. When at last your moment with the busy doctor arrives, you rush through a jumble of symptoms and fears. The doctor interrupts frequently, draws conclusions quickly, examines you briefly, offers advice, and writes a prescription. Out on the street a few minutes later, you're not sure you got your real concerns across.

Rehearsing Your Symptoms

To help recast the central part of that ego-deflating experience—your time with the doctor—prepare in advance. First of all, bring a list of your symptoms. Write down only the main ones, since many doctors get impatient when confronted with a long shopping list. And don't go into detail: The list should serve as a reminder, not a script.

To diagnose your problem, however, the doctor will need a detailed verbal description of your symptoms. So before your appointment, think about them carefully. Take pain, for example. Is it burning, cramping, crushing, cutting, dull, shooting, or throbbing? Does it "radiate" from one site to another? On a scale of 1 to 10, how severe is it?

Does eating, moving, breathing deeply, or anything else make your symptoms better or worse? Do your symptoms interfere with anything you do? Are they steady or do they come and go? If they come and go, how often do they strike and how long do they last? Do they get better or worse at different times of day? Recall when they started, what might have started them, and whether you've had them before.

Rehearsing Your History

Your doctor may not allot much time for a routine office visit. More time is usually scheduled for a first visit or for a comprehensive physical exam, but there'll be more ground to cover.

For a complete physical, be prepared to update your physician on what's happened since your previous exam. If you're a new patient, the doctor will take a complete history. That includes your past illnesses, hospitalizations, and operations, plus health histories of family members. It also includes drug and other allergies; personal habits such as smoking, drinking, and exercising; and work exposure to health hazards. Next, the doctor will ask about current or past problems with each of the major areas of your body, including your heart, lungs, stomach, bowels, bones, joints, muscles, nerves, and skin.

To relay all that information accurately, you'll need to go over it beforehand or perhaps jot down notes. Bring any medical records you've kept. And don't rely on memory for naming your medications and their dosages—bring a list or, better yet, bring the drugs.

Presenting Your Concerns

It's not enough to have the facts; you also have to think about how to present them properly. The wrong emphasis can mislead the doctor and obscure the real problem.

Don't lead off with minor complaints and build up to the main one. The doctor may well place greatest importance on what you mention first.

Symptoms are often rooted in anxiety, depression, or fears about dreaded diseases. (The week after comedienne Gilda Radner died of ovarian cancer, I saw several women with lower-abdominal complaints. Their symptoms disappeared after the exam when I reassured them that their ovaries were normal.) Some doctors may be overly tuned in to possible psychological causes. Occasionally, that can lead them to search for physical causes less thoroughly than they otherwise would. So try not to convey any hint that your symptoms may have emotional roots. Don't minimize or apologize about something that's bothering you. Otherwise, your doctor may be inclined to do the same.

After the doctor has examined you, however, it's important to bring up any fears about what your symptoms mean. If you think a brain tumor may be causing your headaches, for example, say so. You may be reassured to learn that headaches are rarely caused by brain tumors. The doctor might even order tests to rule out that remote possibility. But if you don't speak up, you'll have to live with your fears.

After making an initial assessment, your doctor may recommend further testing or a treatment plan.

⬜ OFFICE VISIT

How to Talk to Your Doctor About Testing

"Were all those tests really necessary?" you may have wondered after leaving your physician's office. As the number and cost of medical tests mount, health-care payers—insurers and the government—are asking the same question. The answer, in many cases, seems to be no.

Physicians used to take great pride in their ability to diagnose illness by simply questioning and examining the patient. They needed only a few simple tests to confirm their impression.

The avalanche of new diagnostic tools has changed all that. It's true that these tools have made diagnosis more accurate. But fancy equipment tends to be used frequently. It's available, it's impressive—and there's a hefty initial investment to recoup. The tendency to order tests increases when third-party payers are footing the bill. It also increases when doctors stand to profit from the tests—for example, if they own a stake in the testing lab.

Many physicians overtest in an effort to rule out every conceivable cause of a patient's complaint. Such zeal may simply reflect extreme diligence. It may also reflect fear of being sued for malpractice for missing a diagnosis.

And it's not just physicians who insist on unnecessary tests. Many patients demand tests to reassure them that nothing is wrong. "Better safe than sorry" is a rationale I often hear. And some patients feel neglected if their doctor fails to order a test that a friend or relative underwent for the same complaint. Physicians usually go along with such demands.

Some Warning Signs

Virtually every test has some potential value, however remote. And the doctor who recommends the test can probably describe that value persuasively. Still, you may be able to avoid some needless tests.

Watch for these two signs of possibly unnecessary testing:

☐ Your doctor keeps repeating tests. It's rarely necessary to check blood tests every week or two, for example, unless the patient is very sick or is taking a drug that requires frequent monitoring.
☐ The tests your doctor orders seem to have nothing to do with your complaint.

If you spot one of these patterns, you can either express your concerns to your doctor or get a second opinion.

What to Ask

To avoid risky, painful, or expensive tests, you'll need information. Start by asking your doctor about the purpose of the test. Then ask about the procedure itself. Will you feel pain or discomfort during or after the test? Will you be exposed to radiation? Can the test cause temporary, permanent, or delayed harm? If so, what are the chances of such harm?

Next, ask about the cost. "It's expensive, but your insurance will cover it" is not an acceptable answer. Take tests because they're necessary, not because someone else is paying.

If the test involves risk or significant discomfort or expense, you'll need to know more about what you stand to gain. Here are some questions to ask:

What are the chances that the test will find something wrong? Those chances increase with the number of risk factors for, or symptoms of, a particular disease. Take sigmoidoscopy—insertion of a lighted, flexible tube into the large intestine to look for colon cancer. If you have no gastrointestinal complaints, the test is not likely to find anything. But if your bowel habits have changed and you have rectal bleeding and a family history of colon cancer, the likelihood of finding disease is much greater.

What would happen if I waited? Suppose an ultrasound test has revealed a small ovarian cyst in a premenopausal woman patient. There's a very small chance that the cyst is cancerous. Her doctor wants to examine the cyst directly, through a surgical incision in her abdomen. The patient asks about delaying that procedure. The doctor says she could wait a few months and repeat the ultrasound to see whether the cyst is growing. If it's not, the cyst probably isn't cancerous. But if it turns out that it is growing, it could be cancerous, and there may be a much smaller chance of successful removal at that point. The patient must then decide whether the prospect of the surgical examination frightens her more than the minute risk of cancer.

Will the test affect treatment? A positive test result should have some practical application: Treatment will be started, stopped, or changed. Satisfying the doctor's or patient's curiosity is rarely a good enough reason to test. If your skin (but not your eyes) has turned yellowish, for example, your doctor may suspect carotenemia— excess carotene, a food pigment, in the blood. But there's little point in testing to confirm that suspicion. No other condition could produce such yellowing in an otherwise healthy person. And carotenemia, caused by a diet high in green and yellow vegetables, is harmless.

Any positive findings that might affect treatment should be confirmed. If a doctor recommends a change in life-style or medication based on a single result, ask to be retested—unless the test is risky or costly.

How reliable is the test? Mammography (breast X rays to detect cancer) is very sensitive in picking up possible abnormalities in women over 35. But it's not as useful in younger women, whose breast tissue is usually denser. Moreover, the risk of breast cancer is very small in women under 35. Those are two reasons against testing a young woman with no symptoms.

Getting Answers

Like other highly trained professionals, most physicians dislike having their knowledge or authority challenged. A defensive or angry doctor may try to pressure you into undergoing a test or may not provide much useful information about it. So confrontation may not gain you much. But if your doctor doesn't answer your reasonable questions in a reasonable manner, you may want to look for another doctor.

Communicating with your doctor will be much easier if you both have similar attitudes toward testing. If you can tolerate some uncertainty—and hate being poked and pricked—find a reliable physician who leans toward clinical judgment. If you like certainty, regardless of what you have to endure to get it, you'll do best with a physician who tests aggressively.

🗌 OFFICE VISIT

When to Fire Your Doctor—and How to Find Another

A 60-year-old attorney, a patient of mine for the past 15 years, sat across the desk from me one morning and said he was leaving my care. "It's not you," he said. "It's just that I can't be kept waiting. My time is just as valuable as yours."

Further discussion was useless. I might have told him about the medical emergencies and other unforeseen problems that can try the patience of those who could reasonably expect me to keep a 10 A.M. appointment sometime before noon. But it would have sounded like an alibi. This man had apparently been kept waiting one time too many. It was clear he had made up his mind.

And he was right. Patients shouldn't tolerate what they see as high-handed or inconsiderate behavior on the part of a doctor—long waits, rushed consultations, perfunctory examinations, brusque or unresponsive answers to questions. Nor should they tolerate a con-descending or authoritarian attitude, or a doctor who blames them when treatment fails. Nor need patients accept without complaint office staff members who are rude, unaccommodating, inattentive, or forgetful.

But don't fire your physician in a moment of anger over an isolated incident. If the relationship has been a long and trusting one, try discussing your grievances. Your doctor may not realize a problem exists. If the problem can be resolved, all to the good. If not, it's time to leave.

There are lots of good doctors, so it's okay to leave a good doctor who's not good for you. And it's absolutely necessary to leave a bad doctor. Don't go back to a doctor who incorrectly diagnoses a sig-nificant problem, prescribes a drug to which you're allergic, fails to follow up an abnormal laboratory result, or makes light of your health complaints.

Starting the Search

How do you find a replacement? There's no sure way to find a personal physician who will meet your needs. But a few measures can help you avoid a poorly qualified physician—and may lead you to the right person.

First you'll need some names. Many people simply ask a friend who seems satisfied with his or her medical care. A better approach, in my view, is to ask a health-care professional—a physician, nurse, therapist, or technician—who has seen the doctor in action. Almost anyone working in a hospital can tell you which doctors are regarded highly by their patients and colleagues.

If you don't know such an insider, call the local hospital and ask the medical staff secretary for the names of several staff physicians. The county medical society can also provide names. Relying on a paid advertisement is a poor way to choose a physician.

Checking Credentials

Once you have the names of a few candidates, investigate their qualifications. Look for a personal physician who's "board certified" in internal medicine or family practice. The specialty boards certify physicians who have completed an approved residency program and passed a test. About half of all internists and almost two-thirds of all family physicians are board certified. A doctor who is "board eligible" has finished an approved residency but has either failed or not yet taken the certifying examination. An internist may also be certified in a subspecialty, such as cardiology or gastroenterology. This may be important to you if you have a particular health problem.

Your new doctor should be affiliated with a hospital accredited by the Joint Commission on Accreditation of Health-Care Organizations. Accredited university and community hospitals routinely check the qualifications and performance of their staff physicians. (You can check a hospital's accreditation by consulting the *American Hospital Association Guide to the Health-Care Field,* available in libraries.) If a physician holds a faculty position at a medical school, so much the better. That means he or she teaches medical students or residents and is probably up-to-date.

Find out where the doctor took his or her residency training. That's more important than the medical school attended. Residency programs at large, typically urban university medical centers tend to provide a wider variety of cases and more hands-on experience than do those at smaller hospitals.

Also find out if the doctor is a fellow of a specialty society, such as the American Academy of Family Physicians or, for internists, the American College of Physicians. Since specialty societies exist mainly to provide continuing education to their members, a doctor's fellowship suggests he or she has some interest in keeping up with the latest research.

How do you get all this information? Consult any of several directories in the library, starting with the American Medical Association's *American Medical Directory,* which is not restricted to AMA members. Board-certified physicians are listed in *Marquis' Directory of Medical Specialists* and the *ABMS* (American Board of Medical Specialties) *Compendium of Certified Medical Specialists.* Note, however, that none of the three directories verifies all information provided by physicians. And some information may be out of date, since the directories are published every other year.

Your county medical society will tell you over the telephone about the credentials that its members have reported. The American Board of Medical Specialties has a toll-free number (800-776-CERT) that will tell you whether a physician is board certified.

Making the Switch

Once you've found a new physician, have your records transferred. Your former physician must honor your written request to forward your records. You needn't feel embarrassed about this. In fact, you might even let your former doctor know why you decided to leave.

Ear Problems

Ringing Ears

Q. *For two years, I've had constant ringing in my ear that's gradually getting stronger. Tests by an ear specialist were inconclusive. What's going on, and what can I do about it?*

A. The cause of ringing or other noise in the ear, called tinnitus, often can't be determined. Tinnitus can result from almost any ear disorder, such as impacted earwax or infection. It can also be a symptom of anemia, cardiovascular disease, or Ménière's disease. Tinnitus is often associated with hearing loss.

Treating the underlying disorder, if one can be found, may stop the noise. If not, you can cover up the noise by playing background music or by using a tinnitus masker, which is worn like a hearing aid and makes a whining sound. Alcohol, caffeine, nicotine, and loud noises may aggravate tinnitus in some people.

Fear of Flying

Q. *I've heard that you shouldn't fly if you have a cold. Is that true?*

A. Not if you take the right precautions. If nasal congestion has blocked the eustachian tube, which connects your nose and middle ear, a change in cabin pressure during takeoff and landing can make the eardrum retract or expand. That can cause pain and possibly even rupture the eardrum.

The risk can be reduced by taking a decongestant—preferably nasal spray or drops—shortly before takeoff. If it's a long flight and congestion recurs, a second dose may be needed about a half hour before landing. Frequent swallowing or yawning can also help. Many flight attendants recommend that passengers place cups containing cotton moistened with hot water over the ears to avoid the ill effects of pressure changes. They swear it works, but no one has studied this remedy.

Ear of Flying

Q. *Whenever I fly, I chew gum and yawn on both ascent and descent. Still, I experience pain in my ears, especially on descent. Afterward, my ears feel like they're "blocked" for the rest of the day. Is there anything I can do about this?*

A. Your problem probably stems from congestion blocking the eustachian tube, which connects your nose and middle ear. When that happens, the change in cabin pressure during takeoff and landing can make the eardrum retract or expand, causing pain and impairing hearing. To keep the eustachian tube open, try taking a decongestant—preferably a short-acting nasal spray or drops, such as phenylephrine 0.5% *(Neo-Synephrine)*—shortly before takeoff. If it's a long flight, a second dose may be needed about a half hour before landing.

Be Still My Beating Heart

Q. *Lately, I've been hearing in my left ear the sound of pulsing blood. The rhythm is the same as my heartbeat. I'm most aware of it when I awaken during the night. Should I be concerned?*

A. Probably not. What you describe is a common disorder known as pulsatile tinnitus. You notice the sound at night simply because your surroundings are quieter then. Your doctor can rule out possible causes, ranging from a buildup of earwax to a partial obstruction in the carotid arteries of the neck. Unless a problem is found, which is unlikely, the pulsatile beat is harmless.

Ménière's Disease

Q. *What can you tell me about Ménière's disease? My doctor says there's no treatment. Is that true?*
A. The cause of Ménière's disease, a disorder that affects the inner ear, is unknown. Symptoms include vertigo (a spinning sensation) and tinnitus (ringing or other noise) in one ear or occasionally both ears. Gradual hearing loss often occurs. An ear, nose, and throat specialist can confirm the diagnosis with tests of balance and hearing. To rule out an acoustic neuroma—a benign tumor that can cause symptoms similar to those of Ménière's disease—a computerized tomography (CT) scan or magnetic resonance image (MRI) of the internal auditory canal within the skull should be done.

Treatment of Ménière's disease is usually not very effective. Strategies include diet therapy (usually low-sodium) and certain medications (antihistamines, sedatives, or diuretics). As a last resort, part of the inner ear may have to be surgically destroyed to provide relief.

Labyrinthitis

Q. *Several months ago, I experienced dizziness so severe that I couldn't walk or even open my eyes. I was rushed to a hospital, where the problem was diagnosed as labyrinthitis and treated with* Antivert. *Four months later, I still sometimes feel light-headed and have trouble keeping my balance when I look back over my shoulder. Will this go on forever?*

A. Probably not. Usually, each succeeding attack gets shorter and milder, although some people continue to have dizzy spells at irregular intervals for many years.

Labyrinthitis is an inflammation of the maze of inner-ear canals that control balance. The disorder usually arises from nasal congestion caused by a cold or allergy. The result is vertigo, a spinning sensation that disrupts balance.

Certain medications may help control the dizziness. These drugs include dimerthydrinate, sold over the counter as *Dramamine,* and meclizine, available by prescription as *Antivert* or over the counter as *Bonine.*

Making a Sound Choice

Q. *My physician suggests I try a hearing aid. Exactly how does a hearing aid work? What should I look for, and what can I expect?*

A. All hearing aids basically consist of a microphone, receiver, amplifier, and battery. And all face the same challenge: to amplify speech without simultaneously amplifying extraneous sounds. Amplified noise can drown out the voice you're trying to hear or just be a major annoyance. No aid can fully restore normal hearing. But new technology is lessening the noise problem.

Most hearing aids are programmed to boost the higher frequencies, which people with hearing problems generally find hardest to pick up, and to suppress the lower frequencies, which predominate in background noise. Customized models tailored to a person's specific pattern of hearing loss are available. So are manually adjustable aids with up to eight degrees of noise suppression. Most sophisticated are computerized hearing aids, which continuously analyze incoming sound and automatically boost or suppress the various frequencies.

Hearing aids come in several different physical designs. From largest to smallest, the major types are:

□ *Body aids*, the old-fashioned kind, which have an earpiece connected by wire to a pocket power pack.
□ *Behind-the-ear aids*, which hook around the back of the ear.
□ *In-the-ear models*, which are molded to fit the depression at the center of the external ear.
□ *In-the-canal devices*, which fit entirely within the ear canal and are barely visible.

A fifth type, eyeglass hearing aids, are built into the frame of the glasses. These are rarely used anymore, since you'd have to do without both hearing aid and eyeglasses whenever the aid was repaired or the eyesight prescription was changed.

Nearly everyone who needs a hearing aid wants a small, inconspicuous device, and many of the newer hearing aids are less conspicuous than ever. But a smaller device isn't right for everyone. People with severe hearing loss generally need the greater power that larger devices offer. Some people have trouble changing the batteries or working the controls on the smaller models. And some need the more complex circuitry that can fit in a larger aid.

An audiologist (nonmedical hearing professional) can help you sift through the numerous options—differences in power, sound quality, ease of operation, adaptability, size, visibility, lifetime of the batteries, price, and warranty features—and can make recommen-

dations based on test results. But only you can make the final decision. Avoid stores with a limited selection, particularly those that
offer only one manufacturer's products. The more models you try,
the better your chance of finding one whose amplification pattern
closely matches your impairment.

It takes time to get used to a hearing aid. And what sounds good
in a store may not sound good in a crowded room or in a strong
wind. So unless you pick a model that's made especially for you, test
it first on a trial or rental basis. And be sure the seller will provide
follow-up care while you're adjusting to the aid.

For further information about hearing loss and hearing aids, call
the Better Hearing Institute's toll-free line (1-800-EAR-WELL). Or
write the Consumer Affairs Department of the American Association of Retired Persons (AARP), 601 E Street N.W., Washington,
DC 20049; 202-434-2277.

The Veterans Administration tests dozens of hearing-aid models
each year, alternating custom-made in-the-ear models one year and
regular models (including on-the-body, over-the-ear, and eyeglass
models) the next. While the VA's top-rated models aren't necessarily best for each individual, the test results can be useful to your
audiologist. You can obtain a summary of the results by writing to
the Audiology and Speech/Language Pathology Service, Veterans
Administration Medical Center, 50 Irving Street N.W., Washington, DC 20422.

🗀 OFFICE VISIT

Hearing Loss: Don't Suffer in Silence

A patient of mine brought her 75-year-old father to see me. He'd
become increasingly withdrawn and seemed depressed. He often
turned down invitations to family get-togethers. When he did come,
he seldom spoke and often seemed to ignore people. And the
little he did say sometimes seemed inappropriate. His daughter
thought he might have Alzheimer's disease. She questioned whether
he should still be living on his own and wanted my opinion about

hiring someone to care for him at home or placing him in a nursing home.

He did seem listless and a bit peculiar. He would answer some of my questions and then not respond at all to others. He never asked me to repeat, but I soon realized that he was hard-of-hearing. He apparently tried to mask the problem by ignoring what he couldn't hear. Some crude hearing tests confirmed the problem; otherwise, the physical exam was normal.

He said he'd realized his hearing was poor but had been ashamed to admit it, fearing that people might treat him like "an old man." Besides, he didn't want a hearing aid. He recalled friends saying that it made things worse by exaggerating noises and producing static.

After a long discussion, I convinced him to try a hearing aid. An otolaryngologist (ear, nose, and throat doctor) ruled out any reversible hearing disorder, and an audiologist (nonmedical hearing professional) fitted him with an aid. Several weeks later, his daughter told me he'd "rejoined the human race."

A Silent Epidemic

Such stories are all too familiar. Close to 30 million Americans—about one in three by age 65—have at least a mild hearing impairment. But people with hearing loss often fail to seek help. Some fear being shunned or patronized for their handicap. Others think that being unable to hear is just another unavoidable burden of aging, or that hearing aids might only compound the problem. Still others are deterred by the cost of the aids, which range from several hundred dollars to $1,500 or more. Only some health insurance plans pay for hearing aids; Medicare doesn't.

Because hearing loss develops gradually, a few people may not notice even a significant impairment. They may attribute their problem to people's mumbling, or dismiss family members' complaints about excessive radio or TV volume as just another form of nagging.

People who can't hear well tend to become isolated. Frustrated by their inability to follow conversations, they may stop trying and simply withdraw. Or they may make puzzling remarks that are unrelated to the conversation. It's easy to mistake such behavior for signs of depression or mental decline.

A Deafening Din

Hearing loss commonly develops as people get older, in part because of the physical deterioration that accompanies aging. Jets, trains, traffic, jackhammers, loudspeakers, and other noisemakers can compound that natural deterioration. Certainly, very loud sounds, such as an explosion, immediately damage the delicate sensory cells of the inner ear. Chronic exposure to any sound that makes conversation difficult, such as the 85 decibels of a food processor, may eventually cause permanent hearing loss.

But noise isn't a threat only to older people. Loud music may be gradually deafening many younger people as well. A numbing 115 decibels—about eight times as loud as the food processor—can pour from the earpieces of a personal stereo. (On the decibel scale, loudness doubles approximately every 10 units.) And rock concerts can be even louder than the headphones—loud enough to do permanent damage in less than half an hour. Indeed, one study found that nearly a third of college freshmen already had detectable signs of hearing loss.

Here are some ways to minimize noise damage:

- ☐ Whenever possible, avoid situations in which you have to raise your voice to carry on a conversation.
- ☐ If someone else can hear the music coming from the headset of your personal stereo, it's too loud.
- ☐ Carry earplugs that you can use when you're exposed to blaring music, roaring motors, or other loud sounds. Inexpensive, compressible foam plugs that expand to fit the ear canal work fairly well. More expensive plastic plugs that an audiologist molds to fit your ear work better. If you're going to be around particularly loud noise, such as the whine of a chain saw, consider wearing an earmuff-style protector.

Detection and Treatment

When hearing deteriorates because of aging or noise, the first sensory cells to go are those that pick up high-frequency sounds. Voices may sound as loud as ever, but certain words become harder to pick up. Since some consonants have a higher frequency than vowels, certain words, such as "shin" and "thin," become difficult to distinguish. Background noise, such as the voices and rattling silverware in a restaurant, can make it particularly difficult to catch what someone is saying. Another early sign that may accompany hearing loss is ringing in the ears.

If you suspect hearing loss, don't just blame it on getting older. See your physician to rule out correctable causes. Earwax, for example, commonly builds up in the ear canal and can significantly reduce hearing. Over-the-counter kits for dissolving earwax may be worth trying, although there's a small chance that the loosened wax will settle deeper in the ear canal. Don't use cotton-tipped applicators, which can tear the ear canal or injure the eardrum. Any hardened wax should be removed by a doctor.

Hearing problems can also be caused by aspirin, the diuretic furosemide *(Lasix)*, nonsteroidal anti-inflammatory drugs such as ibuprofen, the heart drug quinidine *(Cardioquin, Quinaglute)*, and other common medications. Reducing the dosage or switching to alternative drugs can help. Some treatable conditions that affect hearing include circulatory disorders, inner-ear infection, hypothyroidism, otosclerosis (immobilization of the tiny bones that transmit sound vibrations), Paget's disease of the bones, and rheumatoid arthritis.

If there's no correctable cause and the problem affects your daily life—making you strain to catch what people are saying around you, over the phone, or at the movies, for example—a hearing aid can help. While today's devices still have drawbacks, they're a big improvement over the clunky, noisy contraptions that people used to wear.

Exercise

Aerobic Cramping

Q. *About 15 minutes into my aerobics class, my calves begin to cramp. Why does that happen, and how can I prevent it?*

A. Aerobic exercises, especially those that involve bouncing, tend to overwork the large muscle in the calf. The cramping problem might be avoided if you varied your exercise routine to stress different muscle groups.

Always be sure to stretch your calves before and after exercising: Stand about two feet from a wall and place your hands against it. Bend one knee and move the other leg out behind you, keeping that heel on the floor. Lean forward until you feel the stretch in your calf. Hold that position for 30 seconds, then repeat with the opposite leg.

You can also help prevent cramps by drinking plenty of water both before and during strenuous workouts.

Aerobic Exercise

Q. *Exactly what is it that makes an exercise "aerobic"?*

A. During aerobic exercises such as swimming, jogging, and cycling, the muscles demand a continuous supply of oxygen to burn the energy stored in their cells. That forces the body to improve its ability to use oxygen; this eventually benefits the lungs and heart by increasing the efficiency of breathing and pumping oxygenated blood.

Although there's no magical level at which aerobic exercise begins to yield that benefit, you'll do your heart and lungs the most good if you stay within your exercise benefit zone. That means keeping your heart rate at 40 to 60 percent of its maximum for at least 20 minutes three times a week. (To find your maximum heart rate, subtract your age from 220.)

Nonaerobic or isometric exercises, such as weight lifting, release energy from muscle cells through biochemical reactions that don't depend on oxygen. Unlike aerobic workouts, nonaerobic exercises can be safely sustained for only a few seconds. Their main benefit is building muscle strength.

Low-Impact Aerobics

Q. *In a recent report on exercise, you said that low-impact aerobic dance routines minimize stress to the joints but aren't as effective as high-impact routines for aerobic conditioning. If you keep your heart rate within your "exercise benefit zone," aren't low-impact aerobics just as good for conditioning?*

A. Yes. But the less-vigorous workout makes it harder to stay within your exercise benefit zone (40 to 60 percent of your maximum heart rate, determined by subtracting your age from 220). Picking up the intensity of the workout by pumping your arms or working out on a slight incline would keep the impact low and raise your heart rate.

Resting Heart Rate

Q. *What is considered a "healthy" resting heart rate for a 47-year-old man, and how much can an exercise program lower that rate?*

A. A normal resting heart rate varies from person to person but is usually between 60 to 80 beats per minute, regardless of age or gender. With exercise and proper aerobic conditioning, however, the resting heart rate can fall between 50 and 60 beats per minute. Highly trained athletes can have a resting heart rate as low as 40 beats per minute.

Resting Heart Rate II

Q. *I've heard that resting heart rate indicates how aerobically fit you are, and that a rate below average means you're in good shape. But when should you take your pulse to determine that rate? Mine normally ranges from the upper fifties after waking to the midsixties later in the day. When I'm tense and under pressure, my heart rate can soar into the upper eighties. Which of these is my resting heart rate?*

A. The best time to determine your resting heart rate is before you get out of bed in the morning (unless you had a nightmare, which could make your pulse race). The resting heart rate for a well-conditioned adult is between 50 and 60 beats per minute. So your particular rate upon waking is admirable—assuming you exercise regularly. If you're not getting much exercise, however, such a low heart rate could be caused by a problem involving the internal rhythmicity of the heart and should be checked.

Rowing Machines

Q. *What are the benefits of exercising on a rowing machine?*

A. Working out on a rowing machine is one of the best ways to exercise your entire body. The sliding seat works your leg muscles, and the rowing action works the muscles in your arms, shoulders, and back. It's excellent for aerobic fitness and for building muscular strength and endurance. Rowing is also a very good way to burn calories and increase flexibility. However, since rowing involves a fair degree of back flexion, those with recurrent back problems should first check with their physician.

Swimming for Strength

Q. *I swim a mile six days a week. I don't kick as hard as I'd like when swimming because it makes my back ache, so I exercise my legs by* *walking 5 miles once a week. Is this an adequate workout for upper- and lower-body strength?*

A. The swimming certainly gives your upper body a terrific workout. However, it tends to do less for your legs, especially if you don't work them hard. You might want to balance your upper- and lower-body workouts by swimming one day and walking the next.

Weight Lifting and Fainting

Q. *While working out with weights, I suddenly felt weak and started sweating from head to toe. I feared a "silent heart attack," but my doctor checked me on a treadmill and said I was okay. What happened? I'd like to avoid a repeat.*

A. You probably performed a so-called Valsalva maneuver when you were lifting weights: If you strain without exhaling, your blood pressure rises and the pulse drops. When you relax—as the weights are lowered—blood pressure can plunge and you're apt to feel faint.

Proper breathing while you're lifting weights is essential. Before lifting, take a deep breath and then slowly exhale as you lift. The same warning applies to the use of weight machines, such as *Nautilus* equipment.

Varicose and Spider Veins

Q. *I've been doing high-impact aerobic exercise for the past 10 years. Now at 43, I've begun to notice both varicose and spider veins in my legs. Could the exercise be to blame?*

A. Probably not. Heredity, repeated pregnancies, and work that requires prolonged standing will all contribute to varicose veins. No one knows what causes spider veins—small, black or blue vessels in the skin of the inner thighs and lower legs. But there's no evidence that jolting exercise has anything to do with either spider or varicose veins. In fact, varicose veins are more common in people who are not physically active.

Eye Care

Contact Lens Infections?

Q. *I recently read that keeping extended-wear contact lenses in place overnight leads to increased risk of infection. I have been keeping my lenses in for a week at a time. Is that unsafe?*

A. It may be. Extended-wear contact lens users are 10 to 15 times more likely than daily-wear users to develop corneal ulcers, which can become infected. In general, the risk increases with the length of time you wear your lenses, beginning with the first night's use. It is much safer to remove contact lenses daily, then clean and sterilize them each night.

Homemade Saline: Safe When Hot

Q. *Is there really any danger in mixing my own saline solution for contact lens use? I make mine once a week.*

A. Homemade saline is safe to use only for heat-disinfecting your lenses. The heat kills any microbes that may contaminate the solution, which has no preservatives. Using homemade saline for other purposes, such as rinsing lenses, has been linked to a rare but severe corneal infection caused by an amoeba. The infection is difficult to treat and can cause blindness in the affected eye. In one study, 21 to 27 infected lens-wearers had made their own saline.

Declining Vision

Q. *When a physician has determined that a 65-year-old patient has macular degeneration, does this mean eventual blindness? How fast does the condition progress, and is any treatment effective in slowing it down? Are there any support groups?*

A. Degeneration of the macula, a small, oval area near the center of the retina, impairs central visual acuity and color vision. The condition generally starts in a relatively benign "dry" form, but in more severe cases progresses to a sight-threatening "wet" form in which abnormal blood vessels under the retina leak, causing fluid to accumulate under the central retina. This process results in distorted images and blind spots accompanied by reduced visual acuity.

Progression of the disease is extremely variable, and the degree of visual loss depends on the location and extent of the damage. When deterioration is severe in both eyes, a person may become "legally blind": Reading is difficult, and driving isn't permitted. But peripheral vision is usually unaffected, and most daily activities can be maintained.

In some cases, laser therapy can halt macular degeneration by sealing leaking blood vessels. Some ophthalmologists recommend zinc supplements to stem the disease, but there is no hard evidence to support this approach.

The Association for Macular Diseases, which has a newsletter and a members' hotline, can inform you about support groups in your area. The address is 210 East 64th Street, New York, NY 10021; 212-605-3719. The Lighthouse National Center for Vision and Aging can also refer you to support groups. Call toll-free: 800-334-5497.

Glaucoma-Drug Safety

Q. *Two years ago my doctor prescribed twice-a-day Betoptic eyedrops for incipient glaucoma. However, I've read that some glaucoma medications can affect the heart or lungs. Is Betoptic one of them?*

A. Betaxolol (*Betoptic*) is one of a group of medications called beta blockers, which interfere with the action of adrenaline (epinephrine). This hormone, produced by the adrenal glands, helps control the heart rate and blood pressure. While all beta blockers can potentially slow the heart or constrict bronchial tubes in the lungs, *Betoptic* seems less likely than others to produce these side effects. However, if you have a history of asthma or congestive heart failure, your physician should monitor you carefully to ensure that the eyedrops do not make your disorder worse.

New Surgery for Cataracts

Q. *What can you tell me about the phacoemulsification technique of cataract removal? My physician says it hasn't proved its reliability. He wants to wait a year or two before using it. What are its advantages over the current method?*

A. In phacoemulsification, a special device is used to liquefy the cataract—the clouded lens of the eye—before removing it through a tiny incision. Phacoemulsification has been growing in popularity among ophthalmologists because the technique is a generally less-traumatic method of removing a cataract than older, conventional methods. The incision heals faster and with fewer complications. However, there are situations where either the cataract or the surrounding ocular structures do not lend themselves to phacoemulsification. You are well advised to allow your ophthalmologist to perform cataract surgery by the method that will probably work best for you.

Off-the-Rack Glasses

Q. *Now that I'm over 40, is there any reason why I shouldn't use ready-to-wear reading glasses?*

A. Go right ahead, if they're comfortable. Store-bought reading glasses are perfectly safe—and they're quite inexpensive. Such glasses work fine for most people with presbyopia (farsightedness due to aging eyes).

However, you may need to switch to customized prescription lenses if you notice signs of eyestrain, such as headaches or tired eyes. Whether or not you need a professional fitting for corrective lenses, you should still have an eye examination every two years or so after age 45 to ensure that your eyes stay healthy.

Spots Before Your Eyes

Q. *For several years, I've noticed small, gray spots in my vision. They don't prevent me from reading or seeing clearly, but they're annoying. My optometrist says there's no cure and not to worry. Should I do anything more about the problem?*

A. Your optometrist may be right, but you should still be evaluated by an ophthalmologist, a medical doctor who has more training in the diagnosis of eye diseases. The spots you describe are probably just harmless "floaters," but they could also signal other problems.

Floaters

Q. *Is there anything that I can do about "floaters," those harmless spots before the eyes?*

A. Try to ignore them. There's no treatment for floaters, which are actually stringy particles that form as the clear gel-like fluid inside the eye degenerates with age. Fortunately, floaters seldom interfere with vision and tend to disappear on their own. However, a sudden increase in their number or size, especially if accompanied by flashes of light, may signal a disorder of the retina, the light-sensitive tissue at the back of the eye. Eyes with such symptoms should be checked promptly by an ophthalmologist.

Twitching

Q. *For the past year, I've been troubled by frequent twitching in my left lower eyelid. Occasionally, the twitch extends down to the corner of my mouth. Eye exams have ruled out any disease, and my ophthalmologist says there's no treatment. Have you any suggestions?*

A. Such tics usually disappear spontaneously over time and generally require no treatment. Be patient. If yours is very annoying, you might seek a consultation with a neurologist.

Plastic Sunglasses

Q. *Your report on sunglasses says that even clear plastic lenses block most ultraviolet light. Does that mean that my clear plastic prescription eyeglasses provide all the UV protection I need?*

A. Probably. Only people who are at high risk of developing eye damage need to wear lenses with a special coating that blocks additional ultraviolet light. This includes people who spend large amounts of time in the sun; those who have had cataracts removed without the insertion of an artificial lens; and those who take certain medications, such as allopurinol (*Lopurin, Zyloprim*), phenothiazine compounds (*Compazine, Thorazine*), psoralen drugs (*Oxsoralen, Trisoralen*), tretinoin (*Retin-A*), or the antibiotics doxycycline or tetracycline.

Although glass lenses also offer some protection against UV rays, people who will be relying on that type of eyeglasses for protection from sunlight should have the lenses specially coated.

Foot and Leg Pains

Bone Spurs

Q. *My foot doctor has advised surgery for painful bone spurs on the top of my feet. But I can't afford to stay off my feet for eight weeks. Would medication, laser treatment, or anything else relieve the pain?*

A. Bone spurs, an overgrowth of bone at or near joints (usually those of the big toe), don't cause pain; shoe pressure on the spurs does. Try wearing roomier shoes, stretch shoes, or extra-depth orthopedic shoes. Putting pads inside your regular shoes may help, so long as the pads don't put more pressure on the spurs. Aspirin or ibuprofen may relieve the pain temporarily, but that's not a long-term solution. Sometimes an injection of a long-acting corticosteroid (*Deltasone, Depo-Medrol*) can provide relief for months.

If these simple measures aren't sufficient, surgery to file down the protuberances may indeed be your best bet. Recovery from surgery rarely takes eight weeks, however. Most people can resume sedentary activities, such as desk work, within a few days and light walking without crutches or a cane in three or four weeks. So far, laser treatment for bone spurs seems to offer no advantage over traditional surgery.

Feet on Fire

Q. *I'm troubled by a severe burning feeling on the soles of both feet. My circulation is normal, and soaking and applying powders have been to no avail. Could this be a symptom of a serious ailment?*

A. A burning sensation on the soles of your feet can arise from any number of causes, from ill-fitting shoes to diabetes. The most serious cause is peripheral neuropathy—damage to the peripheral nerves—often from diabetes or alcoholism and less commonly from vitamin deficiencies or lead poisoning. A rare disorder called erythromelalgia increases blood flow to the hands and feet and can also produce a searing sensation.

Some people experience fiery feet because they're sensitive to a chemical in the inner lining of their shoes (particularly some types of athletic shoes). Try changing your footgear to see if the problem subsides. If not, see your physician to rule out medical causes.

Morton's Neuroma

Q. *In your report on foot problems, you didn't mention one that has plagued me, Morton's neuroma. What can you tell me about it?*

A. Morton's neuroma, a fairly common abnormality, is a benign tumor of a nerve in the web between two toes. The tumor causes pain when you walk or otherwise put pressure on the area. It may even feel as if a marble or pebble were inside the ball of the foot.

Treatment of the neuroma typically begins with injections of anesthetics or corticosteroids. Orthotics, special shoe inserts, can also help. If these measures don't work, surgical removal of the neuroma usually brings complete relief.

Spare the Scalpel

Q. *I'm 72 years old and have a hammertoe and bunions on both feet. I'm in no pain whatever, but my podiatrist insists that I need surgery to correct the problems. What do you advise?*

A. You should change podiatrists. If the hammertoes and bunions don't bother you and don't hinder your mobility, then surgery is unnecessary.

Spinal Stenosis

Q. *For some time, I've had painful tingling in my legs, especially when I walk. My doctor says that's due to stenosis in my lower spine. What is that, and what can be done about it?*

A. As people get older, spinal stenosis—narrowing of the spinal canal—may begin to develop. Usually the canal becomes crowded due to the growth of bony spurs, a form of osteoarthritis. Less often, displaced joints and ligaments encroach on the spinal canal.

As the canal narrows, it can compress the spinal cord or the nerves that branch from it. That causes symptoms such as yours, as well as weakness and pain. For mild symptoms, nonsurgical treatments may provide adequate relief. These treatments include aspirin, ibuprofen, or other nonsteroidal anti-inflammatory drugs; a spinal brace; and modified posture—leaning forward slightly whenever possible to decrease the pressure on the nerves.

Although those measures don't always work, they're worth trying before resorting to surgery. If necessary, a surgeon can remove parts of the vertebrae and anything else encroaching on the canal. Rehabilitation after the operation can take a while, but most patients eventually report good results.

Treating Swollen Legs

Q. *I've had lymphedema in both legs for 12 years, and my ability to walk has steadily worsened. My doctor's only recommendation is an extremity pump to pressurize a sleeve that covers each leg. Are there any other treatments?*

A. Lymphedema is swelling of an arm or leg due to obstruction of the flow of lymph, a milky-looking body fluid. Leg swelling from lymphedema can be treated in several ways, but all treatments lose effectiveness over time. The "lymph pump" you describe can provide temporary relief early on, when fluid accumulation is less severe. The primary treatment for lymphedema remains the use of good elastic stockings. Various surgical procedures have been tried, generally with little lasting benefit.

Waterlogged Legs

Q. *I am a 75-year-old woman. Last year my feet and legs became so swollen that I couldn't get into my shoes. My doctor said I had "water retention" and gave me a seven-day supply of Maxzide [triamterene and hydrochlorothiazide], which eventually relieved the swelling. What causes water retention, and how can I avoid it?*

A. There are several reasons for leg swelling. One of the most common is varicose veins, in which damage to valves in the large veins of the legs hinders the return of blood to the heart. Blood plasma, which is mostly water, pools in nearby tissue, causing swelling of the legs and feet. Excess dietary salt, sitting or standing for long periods, and hot weather can aggravate the swelling. Exercise such as walking or cycling helps. So does resting with your legs elevated.

Water retention can also be caused by more serious problems, such as heart, liver, and kidney disorders. A medical checkup to rule those out would be wise.

Hair Care

Hair Today, Gone Tomorrow

Q. *Is there a safe way to remove unwanted hair permanently?*

A. Electrolysis is the only technique for permanent hair removal. A fine needle inserted into the hair follicle delivers an electrical impulse that kills the hair root.

Even the most skillful electrologist can have problems with the technique. Applying too much electrical stimulation can scar the tissue around the hair follicle. Too little can fail to destroy the root. Rather than risk scarring, it's better to err on the side of under-stimulation and repeat the procedure, if necessary. However, doing so can become a prolonged, expensive process.

Hair-Loss Help

Q. *My hairline is receding. Can any treatment successfully grow new hair or stop hair loss? Specifically, what can you tell me about* The Helsinki Formula?

A. *The Helsinki Formula* is one of many dubious and unproven hair growth products. The only treatment that does anything at all for hair loss is minoxidil *(Rogaine)*, a prescription medication that is applied to the scalp. But minoxidil works in only about 40 percent of the men treated, and even that estimate may be overoptimistic; it usually produces only moderate regrowth on the crown. Moreover, men who fare the best tend to be younger, recently balding, and to still have some hair in the affected area. Typically, significant results occur only after several months of treatment. In clinical trials the drug has never been shown to restore a receding hairline. Even when it is effective, minoxidil works only as long as it's used: New hair produced by minoxidil sheds within a few months of discontinuation. And using this medication for a lifetime is an expensive proposition. A month's supply costs about $50.

☐ OFFICE VISIT

When Women Lose Their Hair

"It started about six months ago, and it's getting worse," a distraught 53-year-old stockbroker told me. "At this rate, I'm afraid I'll go bald in a year."

She had every reason to be upset. In a culture that worships a full head of "luxurious" hair, it's understandable that hair loss can be accompanied by a sense of emotional loss as well—especially for women. A balding man, at least, has plenty of company; a woman who's losing her hair may feel abnormal. According to a recent poll, about two-thirds of women who are experiencing hair loss say they feel less sexually attractive, compared with about one-third of men. And while a third of these men do nothing special to try to hide their hair loss, virtually all of the women do try.

Some hair loss is inevitable. But when a woman loses more hair than is typical for her age, there is often an underlying cause that can be corrected—or that will correct itself. If hair loss can't be reversed, you can still take steps to minimize the loss.

The Root of Hair Loss

To determine whether you're really losing hair faster than normal, count the hairs you lose during bathing and brushing every day for a week. (Use a strainer over the tub drain, and brush your hair over the sink.) The typical adult sheds about 100 hairs a day. If you consistently find many more than that, you probably are losing ground.

Every hair follicle goes through a cycle: It grows a hair for two to five years, rests for up to six months, sheds the old hair, and starts on a new one. Ordinarily, about 90 percent of the follicles are growing hair at any given time. Anything that shortens the growing phase or prolongs the resting phase will cause gradual hair loss until a new balance is achieved.

Many factors can upset this delicate balance. The most common factor involves hormones and heredity: In some people, the hair follicle in the scalp shuts down in response to male hormones. That response can cause both male- and female-pattern baldness. In men, the hairline typically recedes around the temples and over the crown. Women tend to lose hair more evenly, without developing actual bald spots.

In women, this hormonal sensitivity often shows up after menopause. As production of the female hormone estrogen declines, the small quantities of male hormones still produced by the ovaries are free to function unopposed. The same phenomenon can occur temporarily after childbirth or when a woman goes off oral contraceptives.

A wide range of disorders can also temporarily disrupt the growth-rest balance. Possibilities include a major illness, such as a heart attack; serious physical trauma, such as an auto accident; malnutrition; anemia; and disorders of the endocrine and thyroid glands. Certain drugs, especially chemotherapy for cancer, can also cause temporary hair loss.

Various other disorders can attack the hair follicle itself, sometimes leading to permanent hair loss. These include diseases that affect the scalp, such as psoriasis, discoid lupus, and fungal and bacterial infections, as well as an autoimmune disorder known as alopecia.

Treating Hair Loss

My patient had already seen a dermatologist. He found no evidence of scalp disease and referred her to me. During my examination, I spotted no other possible underlying disorder.

I did learn that this patient had begun menopause about a year before. So her hair loss might have been caused by declining estrogen and a hereditary sensitivity to male hormones. If so, estrogen replacement therapy could have helped reverse the problem. But while such hormone therapy is warranted for women at risk of osteoporosis or coronary heart disease, thinning hair alone doesn't justify that treatment.

I told my patient that she could wait a few months to see if her hair stopped thinning, or she could try to regrow some of her lost hair by using minoxidil. Sold under the brand name *Rogaine*, this prescription drug is the only product approved by the FDA for treating hair loss. It comes in a lotion that you apply directly to your scalp twice a day.

But using minoxidil means making a heavy bet on a long shot. In clinical studies, only about one in eight women who used minoxidil experienced what was generously judged "moderate" growth. It can take up to a year for any new hair to be visible. If it works, you must use it indefinitely at an annual cost of $600. In some people, the drug causes itching and skin irritation.

And that's the approved treatment. None of the many over-the-counter remedies that have sprung up over the years has been shown to grow any hair at all. So they've been declared illegal, though enforcement is difficult. Bogus remedies to avoid include vitamins and other supplements, hair tonics, electric massagers and other devices, and anything else you might come across in the back pages of pulp magazines.

Surgical hair transplants are one rather drastic way to get hair to grow where it otherwise wouldn't—for example, where the follicles have been destroyed by scalp disease. The procedure involves moving small patches of scalp with healthy follicles to balding sites. That can be effective for male-pattern baldness. But it's harder to get good results in women, whose hair loss tends to be more diffuse.

Hair transplants can run as high as $15,000, and they're usually not covered by medical insurance. The whole process can take a year or two to complete, and it's painful. I recommend a high-quality hairpiece instead. While a good wig can cost up to $2,000, it's painless and the results are immediate.

Hold on to Your Hair

My patient decided not to gamble on minoxidil. Within a few months, the thinning stopped on its own. Meanwhile, I had given her some suggestions on how to treat her hair more gently.

Whether or not you're troubled by hair loss, here's how to safeguard what hair you've got:

- ☐ *Don't pull your hair.* When washing, don't massage your scalp vigorously. Dry your hair gently with a towel, or let it dry naturally. Avoid brushes or combs that pull your hair, and don't brush vigorously or any longer than you must.
- ☐ *Don't heat your hair.* Heat can weaken the hair shaft and even damage the follicle. Avoid hot rollers and curling irons. If you use a blow dryer, set it on low heat. Use a hat to protect your hair and scalp from the sun.
- ☐ *Don't use chemicals.* Anything that dries the hair weakens it. So don't color, bleach, or perm your hair. Wear a swimming cap to hold off pool chemicals.
- ☐ *Don't go on a crash diet.* That can result in malnutrition and throw off the growth-rest cycle.

Headaches

Headaches—What to Do and When to Worry

"I've been getting headaches ever since I was in college. I used to get them when I was under pressure—exams, job interviews—but for the last two years, I've had them almost every day."

My patient, a 39-year-old editor, said she'd given up on aspirin and other over-the-counter pain relievers, and now relied on a prescription drug containing codeine. "It's been helping less and less, but I'm afraid I couldn't bear the pain without it." She added that no one seemed to take her seriously. "All they do is give me medications."

I often see patients with similar stories. About three-fourths of adults—women more often than men—have repeated headaches at some point in their lives. About half of all adults get severe headaches. Each year, headaches drive about 42 million Americans to their doctors, making headaches the seventh most common reason for office visits.

In one study, almost a third of headache patients expected total pain relief from their doctors. That's not realistic: Headaches that don't respond to over-the-counter pain relievers (acetaminophen, aspirin, or ibuprofen) may resist prescription drugs as well.

Aching Muscles

Most headaches are tension headaches caused by muscle spasm in the back of the head and neck. In some people, those headaches are virtually continuous for years at a time. The spasm can be sparked by emotional stress or by holding the head in a fixed position (for example, while facing a computer screen or driving for hours).

Sometimes, the pain can be severe. You'd usually feel it in the back of your head, but it could encircle the head in a viselike band.

Tension headaches are sometimes helped by measures to relax the tight muscles. These include massage, hot showers, and heating pads on the back of the neck (some people respond better to cold packs). Biofeedback and muscle-relaxation training may be helpful. And some people find relief with other nontraditional techniques such as acupuncture, hypnosis, or meditation.

Nonprescription pain relievers often help occasional tension headaches. If not, prescription analgesics may do the trick. These include aspirin with codeine *(Empirin with Codeine)*; acetaminophen with codeine *(Tylenol with Codeine)*; aspirin, caffeine, and butalbital *(Fiorinal)*; and aspirin and oxycodone *(Percodan)*.

But for chronic tension headaches, even prescription analgesics aren't always useful. They tend to lose their effectiveness, encourage dependency, and even cause "rebound" headaches when they wear off.

A less addictive, often more effective alternative is a tricyclic antidepressant such as amitriptyline *(Elavil)* or imipramine *(Tofranil)*, which can affect the pain pathways in the brain. A tricyclic must be used for several weeks before it takes effect. Since much lower doses of the antidepressant are needed for pain than for depression, there are generally few or no side effects.

Throbbing Vessels

Much less common than the tension headache is the vascular headache. This kind occurs when the blood vessels on the surface of the brain widen excessively. Your head then literally throbs with pain. A few possible causes include severe hypertension, excessive alcohol consumption, certain medications (such as nitroglycerin for angina), and caffeine withdrawal. Vascular headaches range from mild hangovers to migraines and savage "cluster" headaches.

Migraines are often accompanied by nausea and vomiting, and frequently affect only one side of the head. In the classic form, the pain follows certain warning signs (the aura), such as flashing lights, blind spots, or tingling or numbness on one side of the body. The aura is always the same for each individual. An "abortive" migraine features the aura without the headache.

Biofeedback and other nontraditional techniques occasionally help prevent, though not relieve, migraines; heat and other muscle-relaxing steps generally don't accomplish either.

Since migraines may be sparked by specific factors, sufferers should keep a headache diary to pinpoint any possible triggers. People have blamed their migraines on alcohol, monosodium glutamate (MSG), nitrites, and a host of other foods and drinks. Birth-control pills, estrogen replacement therapy, menstruation, irregular eating and sleeping schedules, and bright lights or noises have also been linked to migraines.

The supposed "migraine personality"—compulsive, neat, and rigid—is probably a myth.

Drugs that constrict blood vessels, notably ergotamine (Ergostat), may relieve migraines if taken at the first sign of the headache. Once a migraine is established, however, the only recourse is to take a narcotic such as meperidine (Demerol) or codeine, head for a darkened room, and try to sleep it off. Recent studies show that nonsteroidal anti-inflammatory agents—such as ibuprofen (Advil, Motrin), indomethacin (Indameth), and others—can alleviate migraines, sometimes as effectively as ergotamine. An experimental drug, sumatriptan, appears to ease migraines about as well as ergotamine, with much milder side effects.

Preventing migraines requires different drugs from those used for relieving the headaches. While neither aspirin nor acetaminophen will relieve migraines, recent research suggests that a regular aspirin regimen may help prevent them. Beta blockers taken daily are often effective—provided side effects, such as lowered pulse or blood pressure, don't develop. Propranolol (Inderal) is the only beta blocker approved for migraines, but others may also help forestall attacks. If you have asthma, don't take beta blockers.

Cluster headaches seldom last for more than an hour or two, but those hours—usually in the middle of the night—can be unbearable. The attacks can occur daily for weeks at a time, and then disappear for long stretches. These headaches usually don't last long enough to be treated effectively. Some sufferers need prescription narcotics.

Danger Signs

Headaches caused by a serious underlying problem—something exerting pressure in or around the brain—are uncommon. Some causes of so-called traction headaches include a bulge in the wall of a blood vessel (aneurysm), an inflamed, swollen artery (arteritis), or an infected, swollen brain membrane (meningitis).

Patients who have severe headaches often fear a brain tumor. But headache is seldom the first indication of a brain tumor. (Other signs, such as seizures, weakness in a limb, or impaired speech or gait, are frequently obvious long before the tumor causes headaches.)

When should you call your doctor about headaches?

- ☐ When they're accompanied by weakness of a limb, loss of balance, or changes in vision or speech.
- ☐ When they're accompanied by nausea and vomiting, fever, or disorientation.
- ☐ When they last longer than 24 hours.
- ☐ When they're severe or frequent, even if they don't last long.
- ☐ When they get worse if you bend over, strain during bowel movements, cough, or have sex.
- ☐ When they get worse over the course of days or weeks.
- ☐ When you've never had such headaches before.

And My Patient?

Careful physical and neurological exams turned up nothing except tight neck muscles. I was sure she had chronic tension headaches. I explained that a normal examination made a serious disorder unlikely. We then discussed tension headaches and the rationales for several treatment options. Since the codeine wasn't helping, I asked her to start giving it up.

Reluctantly, she abandoned her medication and steeled herself for the worst. But the headaches got no worse. Heartened, she tried the tricyclic antidepressant I prescribed and enrolled herself in a biofeedback class. Two months later, she told me that she was much less worried and was having fewer, milder headaches. We began making plans for eventually tapering off the antidepressant.

Health Fears and Risks

Alarm over Smoke Detectors

Q. *The smoke detectors in my house have small print indicating they contain radioactive material. Is there any cause for concern?*

A. No. Ionization detectors use a tiny amount of americium 241, a radioactive element, to make the air in a small chamber conduct an electric current. Smoke particles entering the chamber disrupt the current, setting off the alarm. The risk from the minute amount of radiation emitted is negligible. Such exposure is roughly equivalent to moving from one apartment to another one on the floor above, and hence that much closer to the sun.

A far greater risk is relying on ionization smoke detectors alone to protect your family. Ionization devices respond quickly to open flames. But a slow, smoldering fire, the more common type of home fire, is better detected by photoelectric units, which rely on a beam of light and a light-sensitive photocell. Moreover, photoelectric detectors are almost as good as ionization detectors in responding to "fast" fires. When *Consumer Reports* last tested smoke detectors, the best performers were either photoelectric units or combination units with both a photoelectric and an ionization sensor.

Fear of Fiberglass

Q. *The fiberglass insulation in my basement ceiling is exposed. Because my wife's throat sometimes feels scratchy when she works in the basement, she won't let the children play there for fear the fiberglass is harmful. Is it?*

A. Probably not in this situation. Studies have shown a possible link between exposure to fiberglass and lung cancer, but only in workers who inhale huge amounts of the fibers for many years during manufacture or installation. Fiberglass insulation that is fixed in place usually doesn't give off airborne particles.

Heat, Humidity, and Health

Q. *I'm concerned about the unhealthy effects of heat and humidity in public places. What are the dangers?*

A. Heatstroke and respiratory infection. The risk of heatstroke becomes significant when the ambient, or external, temperature rises above 93°F. The risk of respiratory infection increases as the relative humidity falls below 20 percent. For health and comfort, ambient temperatures of 65° to 75°F and humidity levels of 30 to 60 percent are ideal.

How Much Nicotine?

Q. *In your quiz on the strength of a smoker's addiction, you say that the package label should list how much nicotine is contained in each cigarette. But my brand carries no information at all on nicotine content. What gives?*

A. Although the tobacco industry is not required by law to list that information, most manufacturers do—on the package or the carton, or in their ads. If you can't find it there, call the Federal Trade Commission's consumer hotline (202-326-2222) and ask for a copy of their tar and nicotine report for cigarettes. You may also be able to get the report from a member of your congressional delegation.

Normal Body Temperature

Q. *My temperature never seems to reach the "normal" level of 98.6°F. In fact, I rarely get a reading much higher than 97.5° or so, unless I'm sick. Is this unusual?*

A. Not at all. The time-honored "normal" oral temperature of 98.6°F represents the average for healthy people, and that number recently was revised downward to 98.2°F. Some perfectly healthy people never break 98.0°. In addition, your normal body temperature can vary, depending in part on the time of day: It's consistently lowest in the morning and highest in the late afternoon or evening. That daily variation can range anywhere from about 0.7° to 2.6°F.

▭ OFFICE VISIT

Subtle Symptoms That Signal Danger

After nearly a year of increasing constipation and several recent episodes of vomiting, a 75-year-old retired fire fighter came to see me at the insistence of his wife. Physical examination revealed a distended abdomen, mild dehydration, and evidence of chronic weight loss. Suspecting colon cancer, I immediately admitted him to the hospital for a further workup.

There, my suspicions were confirmed: A tumor had completely encircled a segment of his intestine, narrowing it to the point that virtually no fecal matter at all was able to pass. Emergency surgery relieved the obstruction. But by then it was too late. The cancer had already spread to his liver. He died six months later.

Ominous, Not Always Obvious

If only he'd known how to read the early warning signs, there would have been a better chance of curing his cancer. But he mistakenly blamed the progressive narrowing of his stools on an enlarged prostate gland, a condition he knew he had. He attributed his increasing constipation to having eaten less of late. And he figured that's why he was losing weight.

Unpleasant symptoms of one sort or another are the body's way of letting you know that something's wrong. Most people don't think twice about calling the doctor when they're in pain, when they're running a high fever, or if they've had fainting spells. Naturally, there's less motivation to seek medical help when you're not uncomfortable or anxious. And indeed, most minor annoyances can be safely ignored. But some subtle symptoms can signal real danger. Here are a few warning signs to watch out for:

☐ *Bowel changes.* Changes in bowel habits can be deceptive. Most people would dismiss an occasional bout of stomach upset, bloating, cramps, or constipation as the result of something they ate. And various foods or temporary changes in eating habits can indeed cause such symptoms.

   However, as in the case of my unfortunate patient, altered bowel habits can also be an early warning sign of colorectal cancer. Ovarian cancer can be heralded by similar symptoms. Basically, any change in bowel habits that recurs frequently, persists, or tends to worsen over a period of several weeks is cause for concern and warrants a visit to the doctor.

☐ *Rectal bleeding.* People with hemorrhoids sometimes pass blood in their stool; so it's easy to dismiss rectal bleeding as just another hemorrhoidal flare-up. But bleeding can also signal benign or malignant polyps, or possibly diverticula—small protrusions of the intestinal wall that sometimes become infected. Whatever the cause—even if it turns out to be nothing more than hemorrhoids—rectal bleeding always deserves medical attention.

☐ *Weight loss.* Most overweight people would probably be happy to lose weight without even trying. But if you lose more weight than can be explained by obvious changes in diet and exercise, that's nothing to celebrate. Such unexplained weight loss can be an early sign of diseases such as diabetes, poor absorption of nutrients from the intestinal tract, or an overactive thyroid gland.

   All those disorders can cause you to lose weight even though you're eating just as much or even more than usual. If you already happen to be dieting, the extra weight loss may be mistaken for a sign of success.

☐ *Night sweats.* This potentially serious symptom can also be easily overlooked, especially if sweating coincides with hot nights in a room that's not air-conditioned. But repeated night sweats deserve a closer look. Sometimes mild but more often drench-ing, these sweats are usually the result of a low-grade fever that breaks out during the night, when body temperature is normally at its lowest. That fever may be the first sign of a chronic infec-tion, such as tuberculosis, AIDS, or an infected heart valve. Or the cause could be certain tumors, such as lymphomas, kidney cancer, or other cancers.

Some women experience night sweats because of hormonal changes in the early stages after menopause. Usually, however, menopausal sweats also occur during the daytime. Although that phenomenon can be embarrassing and uncomfortable, it's not a sign of trouble; if necessary, a course of estrogen replace-ment therapy can relieve the problem.

☐ *Hoarseness.* If you abuse your voice, you'll make yourself hoarse. It's easy to ignore that minor annoyance, especially if you can find a reason for it—like yelling at the kids, cheering at a ball game, or campaigning for political office. A lingering cold can also leave you hoarse for a while.

But if hoarseness persists longer than a few weeks, especially if you're a smoker, there could be something more to it and you should see a doctor. Blood tests will rule out an under-active thyroid gland, which can cause thickening of the vocal cords and subsequent hoarseness. To check for benign polyps on the vocal cords or for throat cancer, a physician will perform a laryngoscopy, a procedure in which a flexible, lighted tube is inserted into the nose and down the back of the throat.

☐ *Leg pains.* Tired, achy legs can be brought on by a long day at the mall. But if even a short walk when you're well rested causes leg pain, it could be something more serious. If the pain is limited to one calf, it could signal narrowing of the blood ves-sels from arteriosclerosis. If you have pain in both legs, it could be the result of spinal stenosis, an overgrowth of bony tissue in the lower spine that compresses the nerves.

☐ *Red stretch marks.* Stretch marks, which are usually found on the abdomen, flanks, and breasts, are permanent signs of rapid weight gain and are often caused by pregnancy. These pale or silvery areas of thinned skin are at worst a cosmetic concern.

But stretch marks that are red or purplish may indicate Cushing's disease, a disorder in which the adrenal glands produce too much of the hormone cortisol, thinning the skin and bones and increasing the risk of infection. Such stretch marks are especially likely to mean Cushing's disease in people who already have a triad of conditions: diabetes, hypertension, and osteoporosis.

When to Call the Doctor

This rundown of seemingly benign symptoms shouldn't frighten you into calling your doctor every time you sneeze. A few rules of thumb can help you decide whether to seek medical attention. A symptom you might be tempted to ignore should be taken seriously if it:

☐ Represents a sudden change from your usual patterns
☐ Persists for more than two or three weeks
☐ Gradually gets worse
☐ Interferes with your daily routine
☐ Seems like an exaggerated version of a familiar symptom you were previously able to explain.

☐ OFFICE VISIT

When Not to Worry

One Sunday morning a few months ago, a telephone call interrupted my leisurely breakfast. The voice belonged to a young man whose family I had known for years. In desperate tones he pleaded with me to meet him at my office.

There, behind closed doors, he confided that he had had intercourse with his girlfriend that morning. Afterward, as he removed the condom, he noticed that his ejaculate was bloody. He was sure he had either AIDS or cancer.

I promptly reassured him that blood in the semen, called hematospermia, is a symptom of neither disease. It usually stems from a tiny blood vessel in the prostate that's ruptured during orgasm. I told him it would probably never happen to him again. If it did recur with his next ejaculation, he might have a mild infection of the prostate, which could be easily treated.

Assume the Best

Hematospermia is just one of several alarming yet medically insignificant conditions. After all, who wouldn't worry when the body suddenly behaves in an unusual or frightening fashion?

I have warned about potentially dangerous symptoms that patients often overlook (see "Subtle Symptoms That Signal Danger," page 156.). More often, it's the harmless things that command attention. Here I'll describe a few common conditions that invariably send patients running to the doctor, when actually all that's needed is minimal attention or simple reassurance. Perhaps knowing this information in advance will spare you needless distress—and maybe the cost of an office visit.

☐ *Red-eye special.* Subconjunctival hemorrhage sounds horrendous and looks even worse. One eye suddenly becomes literally blood-red due to a leaky blood vessel in the conjunctiva, the delicate transparent membrane that covers the whites of the eyes. That can be caused by just about any effort that temporarily increases pressure in the head—coughing, sneezing, bending over, lifting weights, straining during a bowel movement, or even orgasm.

Despite its appearance, subconjunctival hemorrhage is painless and harmless, and it never interferes with vision. The blood is slowly reabsorbed and disappears over the next few weeks. While you're waiting, tinted glasses can help make the problem less conspicuous.

☐ *Discolored skin.* You might be upset if you noticed your skin turning an orangy shade of yellow. Could it be jaundice (the result of excess bile in the blood) due to hepatitis or some other disease? Not if the whites of your eyes aren't turning yellow, too. More likely the discoloration just means you've been eating lots of carrots or taking beta-carotene supplements.

Carotenemia is the medical term for increased blood levels of carotene, a vitamin-A precursor found mainly in fruits and vegetables, especially carrots and sweet potatoes. The excess carotene is deposited in the skin, where it imparts that distinctive color. Aside from lending the appearance of a bad tan, high blood levels of carotene are harmless; enzymes in the body limit the nutrient's conversion to vitamin A so the vitamin doesn't reach toxic levels. If you don't like the color, cut down on the carrots or supplements. Your skin will return to normal after a few weeks.

☐ *Nocturnal leg cramps* can be quite painful. But they're rarely associated with a serious medical problem. Most often, nighttime leg cramps are the delayed result of strenuous activity during the day. Paradoxically, however, they can also result from inactivity. So the first step in remedying the cramps is to adjust your daytime activity one way or the other. Beyond that, try daily calf-stretching exercises, especially just before going to bed. Quinine sulfate tablets, available over the counter, can also reduce the frequency of cramps.

If you are stricken, it's important to "break" the cramp as quickly as possible: An attack that's allowed to go on for more than a minute or so will leave that calf aching for several days afterward. That lingering pain can sometimes be confused with phlebitis, an inflamed vein obstructed by blood clots; at that point, you'd need professional evaluation to make the distinction. To break the cramp, stretch your leg out straight and forcibly bend your toes back toward your nose.

☐ *"Sighing respirations,"* a type of abnormal breathing, often causes a great deal of anxiety. Ironically, the condition is caused by underlying anxiety in the first place. Although it can be worrisome to the sufferer, the problem has nothing to do with the lungs.

Typically, the patient complains of a frustrated effort to inhale deeply. It's as if you had been interrupted halfway through a yawn. The distressing sensation may occur several times an hour. Meanwhile, tests of pulmonary function and breathing rhythm will detect nothing at all.

Since sighing respirations thrive on anxiety, they often sub-side once the patient has been reassured that there's no med-ical problem. If they don't go away, the underlying anxiety should be treated through psychotherapy and possibly medi-cation.

☐ *Low blood pressure.* Patients sometimes seek advice because they're worried that their blood pressure is too low. They may have had their readings taken at the local supermarket or tried out a relative's home monitor. In fact, many perfectly healthy people—especially short, slim women—have systolic readings (the higher number) of less than 100 mm/Hg. So long as you're feeling fine and don't get light-headed when you arise from a lying or sitting position, your "low blood pressure" is no cause for concern. To the contrary, it's good for the cardiovascular system, since it puts less stress on the blood vessels.

☐ *Painful breastbone.* I often see patients who are troubled by this mysterious syndrome, especially during the summer months or after they return from a tropical vacation in the winter. Out of nowhere, it seems, a painful lump develops at the lower end of the breastbone. Actually, the "lump" is just normal cartilage that's suddenly become noticeable only because it's sore. The victim has invariably been lying belly down for long, relaxing hours on the sand. The sensitivity subsides within a few days after avoiding that beach position.

Ignorance Is Not Bliss

Perhaps feeling somewhat sheepish as he left my office, my young patient was nevertheless much relieved to know that his fears were unfounded. When I spoke with him a few weeks later, he had had no further episodes. I doubt he ever will. But if he does, his new understanding should spare him some grief.

While it's still a good idea at least to call your physician the first time unusual signs or symptoms develop, don't assume the worst. Oftentimes, reassurance is the only treatment that's needed.

▭ OFFICE VISIT

How to Make Sense of Medical News

Last year, a 48-year-old college professor came to see me about increasingly severe headaches that had struck early each morning for two weeks. "I think I know what's wrong," he said. "The headaches started right after I stopped taking my medication."

I had prescribed a diuretic six years earlier to control his hypertension. Without the drug, his blood pressure had now soared to a distressing 180 over 110. Why had he stopped following my prescription?

"I saw a headline two weeks ago that scared me. It said diuretics could boost my chance of having a heart attack."

Unless a medication is causing severe side effects, stopping it without first talking to your physician can be disastrous. But my patient might not have abandoned his medication if he'd read that news story with a critical eye. He might have noticed, for example, that the study was partly funded by the maker of a competing antihypertensive drug. Such a study may be less credible than one financed by an independent nonprofit foundation or a government agency.

He might also have noticed that the news story described a rise in blood-cholesterol levels, not in actual heart attacks.

Most important, he might have seen that the subjects took the drug for only four months—not long enough to establish that the cholesterol rise would be permanent. Indeed, several previous studies lasting a year or more had found that the rise does not persist. But the news story never mentioned those studies—or any other research on diuretics and cholesterol.

Not only do news reports sometimes fail to mention all the relevant facts, they don't always get the facts they do mention right. In this case, the newspaper incorrectly reported that cholesterol levels climbed an average of 15 percent, rather than the actual 5 percent.

The Critical Reader

Whenever you read or hear about a new study, try putting it in perspective. Ask yourself these questions:

☐ Does the news report mention any other studies that support the current findings? A single, uncorroborated study seldom constitutes strong evidence of anything, one way or the other.

☐ What were the age and sex of the subjects? If yours are different from theirs, the results may not apply to you.

☐ Did the story describe the study design? If not, don't trust the findings. You can't judge their validity without knowing how they were obtained.

These design features tend to increase a study's validity:

Human subjects rather than animals or tissue in a test tube.

Large number of subjects.

Long duration of treatment and follow-up.

A *control group* consisting of untreated subjects similar to those in the treatment group. That lets researchers figure out whether any apparent effects of treatment might actually have occurred by chance.

Random assignment of subjects to the treatment or no-treatment group. That helps ensure that the two groups are identical before testing starts.

A *placebo,* or dummy treatment, given to the control subjects. That keeps them from knowing whether they're getting treatment, a realization that can create self-fulfilling expectations.

Double-blind design, in which researchers as well as subjects are kept in the dark about who is receiving the drug and who is getting the placebo. Knowing who got what could bias the way researchers collect and interpret data.

Prospective rather than retrospective design. Prospective studies follow subjects from the start of the study to some point in the future. Retrospective studies look back on what happened to subjects in the past. Since prospective studies are specifically designed to gather new data on the topic at hand, they tend to be more reliable than retrospective studies, which rely on other people's records and recollections. (Prospective studies are usually interventional, with subjects randomly assigned to groups, whereas retrospective studies are always observational.)

Is It For You?

Even if a finding is valid and backed by other studies, it may not warrant changing your habits or your treatment. The risks of a new drug, for example, may not be immediately clear, since the full spectrum of possible side effects becomes evident only after years of widespread clinical use.

Moreover, a drug can be reasonably safe and effective for most people but not for you. Two months ago, a patient with congestive heart failure called me to demand that I switch him to enalapril, an ACE inhibitor. That morning, a headline in *The New York Times* had proclaimed: "Studies Find Drug Cuts Heart Failure Deaths."

Since I read *The Times* over breakfast each morning, I had seen the story. The research seemed to be sound. But enalapril can hamper kidney function. And this patient already had kidney problems. Despite the drug's potential benefits, it was too risky for him.

Even a family history of certain medical problems can make a drug inappropriate. So can another medication you're taking, or a personal habit such as smoking or drinking. Those could interact with the drug, making it less effective or more hazardous than the headlines suggest.

To find out whether a drug you've read or heard about is right for you, get the information you need to make that individual choice: Look it up in the United States Pharmacopeia's *Complete Drug Reference* (available in most libraries, or from Consumer Reports Books), which lists side effects and contraindications of prescription drugs. If the drug still seems appropriate, talk to your doctor.

Hepatitis

Enter Hepatitis C

Q. *My physician has determined that I have non-A, non-B hepatitis. He also says there's no effective treatment. Can you add anything to this?*

A. You probably have hepatitis C. A recently developed test now allows doctors to hang this diagnosis on most people previously said to have non-A, non-B hepatitis.

The hepatitis C virus is transmitted primarily through blood transfusions or infected intravenous drug needles, but it may also be contracted through sexual activity. Chronic liver disease develops in about half of those infected and may last for years without causing symptoms. Significant liver damage occurs in about 20 percent of those with the chronic form of the disease.

The most common course of action for the hepatitis C patient is to monitor liver function periodically by blood tests. If the tests show no progressive impairment, no treatment is necessary. If the tests indicate that liver function is worsening, a biopsy of the liver may determine if treatment is appropriate. A new drug—interferon alpha—has shown favorable results in approximately half the patients treated, but the benefits tend to disappear when treatment is stopped.

More on Hepatitis C

Q. *I'm a 44-year-old woman in apparent good health and have never had a blood transfusion or taken intravenous drugs. But six months ago, when I donated blood, the Red Cross notified me that I'd tested positive for hepatitis C antibodies. Should I be concerned?*

A. Hepatitis C is well known to be transmitted through the blood and through sexual contact but may be transmitted in other ways as well. The test you took implies prior infection with this virus, but it doesn't tell if you have active hepatitis. (It can take a full six months after infection for antibodies to appear in the blood-stream.) Since it's possible to have low-grade hepatitis without symptoms, you should have liver-function tests now and periodically in the future.

Hernias

Lasers for Hernia Repair

Q. *I expect to need surgery for a hernia. Is the new laser technique better than a conventional operation?*

A. No. When part of the intestine "herniates" through the muscles of the abdominal wall, a surgeon must reposition the herniated segment and reinforce the weakened muscle. But the incision is the same whether the surgeon uses a scalpel or a laser. Both procedures are performed under local anesthesia on an outpatient basis. Some surgeons use lasers to "weld" the wall of the abdomen shut; but that weak bond still has to be reinforced by sutures, and the method won't make you heal any faster.

Consumers Union's medical consultants believe that conventional surgery is the best way to repair a hernia.

Umbilical Rupture

Q. *My 48-year-old husband's doctor recommends surgical repair for an umbilical rupture. But it's not causing any discomfort now, and other doctors never noticed it. Is surgery really necessary?*

A. Perhaps not. An umbilical (belly button) rupture, or hernia, is caused by weakness or separation of the abdominal muscle fibers near the navel. When you stand, cough, or strain, the hernia becomes apparent: A portion of the intestine pushes through the muscle and appears as a bulge under the skin. Most of the time, the intestine can be put back into place if the person lies down and gently presses against the bulge. Such hernias are usually congenital but may not be detected until middle age.

Surgery can prevent "strangulation"—impaired blood flow to a trapped portion of intestine—but strangulation isn't likely anyway. If your husband remains free of pain and the bulge doesn't bother him, he may be able to do without an operation. However, if pain develops, he should return to his physician and reconsider surgery.

⬜ Herpes Simplex

Cold Sores

Q. *I'm now 80 years old and have had outbreaks of fever blisters on my lips, nose, and chin for most of my life. What's the best way to control these painful sores?*

A. The only effective treatment for herpes simplex virus type 1 (also known as fever blisters or cold sores) is the prescription anti-viral drug acyclovir *(Zovirax)*. At the first sign of an outbreak, apply the ointment several times a day for about a week. (The capsule form is not effective against herpes simplex type 1.) Topical acyclovir won't cure herpes simplex, but it may help relieve the pain and help heal the sores, if any.

Herpes Treatment

Q. *Has any progress been made against genital herpes [herpes simplex virus type 2] since Zovirax was introduced in the 1980s?*

A. Not much. Acyclovir (*Zovirax*) is still the treatment of choice for people who have more than six episodes of genital herpes per year. Taking acyclovir every day as a preventive measure can decrease the severity of symptoms and the frequency of recurrences. Unfortunately, there's no cure in sight. Recent tests of an experimental vaccine were disappointing.

Cold Sores and Shingles?

Q. *I have recurring cold sores on my mouth and chin. I've heard that the herpes simplex virus that causes them is related to the virus that causes shingles. Does that mean I'm more likely to get shingles eventually?*

A. No. Shingles, also known as herpes zoster, is caused by the varicella zoster virus, the same virus that causes chicken pox. Although the skin lesions of the herpes simplex virus are similar to those caused by the varicella zoster virus, the two viruses are still quite distinct. It's not known why the varicella zoster virus resurfaces years later as shingles in up to 20 percent of people who have had chicken pox—but it's not because they have cold sores.

Hypoglycemia

Five-Hour Glucose-Tolerance Test

Q. *I've read different things about the five-hour glucose-tolerance test for hypoglycemia. Is the test valid?*

A. No. In the 1970s, practitioners using the test incorrectly diagnosed many people as having hypoglycemia (low blood sugar). The test measures blood-sugar levels in individuals after they drink a measured dose of glucose. Readings are taken every hour for five hours. But in many perfectly healthy people, especially women, sugar levels routinely dip into the hypoglycemic range during the fourth or fifth hour. So the results are meaningless.

To diagnose hypoglycemia, blood for sugar analysis should be drawn *while* symptoms are occurring. (Symptoms include sweating, nervousness, heart palpitations, muscle tremors, visual disturbances, headaches, faintness, and confusion.) If that sugar level is really low, more tests must be done to pinpoint the cause.

Immunizations

Adult Immunizations

Q. *How often do adults need to have a tetanus shot or any other routine shots?*

A. All adults should receive a tetanus-diptheria toxoid booster every 10 years. If an injury that might lead to tetanus occurs more than five years after the last shot, another booster should be given. (The next shot would then be given 10 years from that date.) People age 65 or over and those in certain high-risk groups should receive pneumococcal vaccine once and influenza vaccine annually.

Just One Shot for Pneumonia?

Q. *You've said that people 65 and older should receive pneumococcal vaccine once. But some doctors have told me they recommend the shot* *every five years. I had one six years ago when I was 71. Should I get another?*

A. Healthy older people generally need only one dose of pneumococcal vaccine. (You should consider a single revaccination with the "23-valent" vaccine if you previously received the older "14-valent" type.) However, if you have a medical condition such as heart, kidney, liver, or lung disease, diabetes, Hodgkin's disease, cerebrospinal fluid leaks, an immune system disorder, or sickle-cell anemia, you could be susceptible to complications from pneumonia. So you should get a shot every six years.

Flu Shots

Q. *I've heard so many opinions, pro and con, about flu shots. Who should get a flu shot? How effective is it? When is the best time to get one?*

A. Anyone who can tolerate a flu shot should consider getting one before the influenza season begins. That's especially important for these high-risk groups:

☐ People age 65 or over.
☐ People with chronic lung or heart disorders, including children with asthma.
☐ Adults and children who during the preceding year needed regular medical care or hospitalization for a chronic disease: diabetes, kidney disorders, sickle-cell disease, or suppressed immune systems (including AIDS).
☐ Children and teenagers 6 months to 18 years who are on long-term aspirin therapy.
☐ People who live with or care for a person at high risk.

A flu shot takes about two weeks to provide protection and lasts about six months. But the injection does not provide full immunity in all cases. It's about 90 percent effective in young, healthy people, and 75 percent effective in elderly, high-risk people—for the strains of influenza included in the vaccine. If an unexpected strain of flu pops up during the flu season, the vaccine may not work at all.

Generally, October is the best time for a flu shot, but any time between September and February is better than not at all. Travelers abroad, however, should consider a flu shot whatever the month. They may risk exposure to the virus at any time of year.

Can You Tolerate a Flu Shot?

Q. *You say that "anyone who can tolerate a flu shot" should consider getting one. Exactly who can't tolerate a flu shot?*

A. People allergic to eggs, which are used to make the influenza vaccine, should not receive the shot. And people with an acute illness, such as a respiratory, gastrointestinal, or urinary-tract infection, should wait until they recover. Pregnant women would be prudent to delay a flu shot until after their first trimester, unless they are at high risk of getting influenza.

☐ Men's Health

Prostate Problems

Q. *Can urinary or sexual habits affect the incidence or severity of an enlarged prostate or any other prostate problems?*

A. Those personal habits have nothing to do with the development of any prostate problems. However, modifying certain habits may help reduce the severity of symptoms. For example, urinating more frequently to keep the bladder from overfilling, allowing enough time to empty the bladder completely, and cutting back on fluids for several hours before bedtime can help reduce symptoms from an enlarged prostate. And since congestion in the prostate gland can aggravate the discomfort from chronic prostatitis (inflammation often due to bacterial infection), many urologists recommend frequent ejaculations to minimize that discomfort.

PSA Test for Prostate Cancer

Q. *I recently read about a blood test for prostate cancer called PSA. How does this test work, and is it effective?*

A. Prostate-specific antigen, or PSA, is a protein made in the prostate gland and released into the bloodstream. The PSA blood test can indeed detect early prostate cancer. But it's often hard to tell whether an elevated reading signals cancer or merely benign enlargement of the prostate gland. Now researchers have found that repeating the PSA test each year can help physicians make this distinction.

Researchers at Johns Hopkins University found that PSA levels remain quite stable (below the "normal" limit of 4.0 micrograms per liter) in healthy men from year to year. In men with a noncancerous enlarged prostate, these levels rise only slightly each year. But cancer causes PSA scores to rise much faster.

The researchers concluded that even if the PSA level remains in the "normal" range, a jump of more than 0.75 microgram in one year is strong evidence of prostate cancer. Since a rapidly rising PSA level could signal a quick-growing tumor, an annual test might also help physicians determine whether immediate treatment is necessary.

Consumers Union's medical consultants recommend that all men age 50 and older have the PSA test as well as a digital rectal exam every year. Because a vigorous finger rectal exam itself may raise PSA levels for as long as a week or two, the blood test should be done first.

High PSA and Prostate Cancer

Q. *My doctor ordered a PSA blood test for prostate cancer during a routine physical exam last fall. The results showed a score of 28, so he ordered a biopsy; it revealed no sign of cancer. I've since had another PSA test, which came out just as high. What, if anything, should I do about it?*

A. Talk to your doctor about having another biopsy—soon. As we reported, a PSA (prostate-specific antigen) score above 10 indicates a strong probability of prostate cancer. (Blood for a PSA test should be drawn *before* any digital examination of the prostate, to avoid a possibly false-elevated score.) The repeat biopsy should be guided by rectal ultrasound, which can help identify any suspicious areas in the prostate.

Blocking Prostate Growth

Q. *I understand that there's a new medication for an enlarged prostate. What can you tell me about it?*

A. An enlarged prostate gland—its medical name is benign prostatic hyperplasia (BPH)—affects more than half of all men over age 50. This noncancerous condition causes urinary symptoms such as a frequent, urgent need to urinate; a delayed, weak, or interrupted urinary stream; and an inability to empty the bladder fully, which can lead to urinary-tract infection and even kidney damage.

A new drug called finasteride (*Proscar*) shrinks the prostate by interfering with production of the hormone that stimulates prostatic growth. Controlled clinical trials involving 1,645 men found that after a year on the drug, about one-third of patients experienced greatly improved urinary flow; another third had at least some relief. Side effects were minimal (about 4 percent), and were limited to sexual dysfunction—impotence, decreased libido, or a decreased volume of ejaculate. It's too soon to know whether long-term use may cause other problems. And finasteride must be taken indefinitely, since prostate growth resumes when treatment stops. A year's supply of the medication costs about $600.

If you're facing surgery for BPH, talk to your physician about trying drug treatment first.

Heating an Enlarged Prostate

Q. *In discussing prostate problems, you didn't mention hyperthermia as an alternative to traditional surgery for an enlarged prostate. Why not?*

A. Because it's not reliable. Hyperthermia (microwave heating) is still in the early experimental stages. So far, the results are not too encouraging. In one trial, the success rate for hyperthermia was even lower than the rate of spontaneous improvement.

Prostate Stones

Q. *I have been diagnosed as having prostate stones. I'm worried that they might increase my chances of getting cancer. Will I pass these stones as kidney stones are sometimes passed?*

A. There's nothing to fear about so-called prostate stones. They're actually just tiny calcium deposits that form where the gland was inflamed at one time. These "stones" can't be passed, and they don't lead to cancer.

Prostatectomy and Infertility

Q. *You recently said that after surgery for an enlarged prostate, virtually all men become infertile due to "retrograde ejaculation," in which semen travels back up into the bladder. Aren't there ways to isolate semen from the urine for artificial insemination?*

A. Yes. But the reliability of those techniques varies from person to person, depending on the viability of the sperm. Men who want to father a child after prostate surgery may also want to consider storing sperm at a sperm bank before the operation. However, that's not a sure bet either, since the freezing and thawing make sperm less vigorous.

Impotence and Blood-Pressure Drugs

Q. *The medication I take for high blood pressure is making me impotent. Is there a drug that can control my blood pressure without affecting my sex life?*

A. Probably not. All of the widely used types of blood-pressure drugs have been associated in varying degrees with impotence. However, two classes of antihypertensive drugs may be less likely to cause impotence. One is a group known as ACE inhibitors, such as captopril (Capoten), enalapril (Vasotec), and lisinopril (Prinivil, Zestril). The other group, called calcium channel blockers, includes such drugs as diltiazem (Cardizem), nicardipine (Cardene), nifedipine (Procardia), and verapamil (Calan, Isoptin). If your current medication can be safely changed to one of these, without compromising blood-pressure control, switching may solve your problem.

Impotence and Hormones

Q. *Six years ago, at age 65, I became impotent and had little sexual desire. Although my testosterone level was normal, I responded to hormone injections. However, my doctor refused to continue them for fear of stimulating latent prostate cancer cells. Now one prominent urologist is offering testosterone, while another says I would be "crazy" to take it. What's the story?*

A. There is no good clinical evidence that testosterone injections can improve potency in men with normal testosterone levels. Your positive reaction to the hormone may have been a placebo effect—a psychological response to taking medication.

The concern that testosterone may stimulate prostate cancer is reasonable. It's based on animal studies: the fact that testosterone accelerates prostate cancer growth, and the observation that prostatic cancer cells are present in a large percentage of aging men.

Advice Gets a C

Q. *Three years ago I underwent prostate surgery. Since then, on the advice of my urologist, I have been taking 500 milligrams of vitamin C twice a day to help prevent infection. Can you comment on this?*

A. The dose of vitamin C you're taking may make your urine somewhat acidic, but you can't count on it to inhibit bacterial growth. In addition, you probably don't need it. Your risk of infection presumably ended when the prostate surgery relieved your urinary obstruction.

Peyronie's Disease

Q. *What can you tell me about Peyronie's disease?*

A. It's a common disorder in men, mainly those who are ages 40 to 60. In Peyronie's disease, fibers on one side of the penis contract. As a result, the penis slowly becomes curved—but so slowly that many men with the disorder aren't even aware that it's happening.

The cause of the disease is unknown and there's no proven medical treatment. Many cases resolve on their own in a year or so. But if scar tissue forms, the penis becomes permanently curved. If the curvature interferes with erections or intercourse, surgery may be necessary to remove the scar tissue.

Vasectomy: Any Risks?

Q. *I am considering having a vasectomy but have heard it can increase the risk of heart attack. Is that true? And are there any other risks associated with a vasectomy?*

A. The purported link between vasectomy and heart disease appeared in a small study conducted more than a decade ago on monkeys. This link has since been discounted by a host of subsequent studies. More recently, two studies proposed a link between vasectomy and prostate cancer. The World Health Organization views any such association as unlikely and advises no change in policy with regard to vasectomy. Further research is needed either to establish or to disprove an association between vasectomy and prostate cancer. Any man who has undergone a vasectomy should have a digital rectal exam and a blood test (prostate-specific antigen) annually beginning at age 50.

⬜ Neurological Problems

Arm Numbness

Q. *I frequently have altered sensation and temperature perception in my right hand and arm. And one or both arms are often numb when I wake. What's the problem?*

A. Numbness or tingling in an arm during sleep is usually caused by pressure on a nerve, not poor circulation as is commonly believed. When one arm is affected, the pressure is often caused by a favorite sleeping position—for example, tucking your hand under your head or pillow. In that case, the numbness would disappear within a minute or two after you relieve the pressure. When the problem strikes both arms or either one during waking hours, you should be evaluated by a physician for other possible disorders, including carpal tunnel syndrome, disk disease of the neck or arthritis of the neck, and thoracic outlet obstruction syndrome.

Hand Tremor

Q. *I've had a slight tremor in my hands for the past two or three years. In recent months it seems to have become more pronounced. Is there anything that can alleviate this condition?*

A. Yes, but the specific treatment depends on the underlying cause. Among the many causes for tremor: an overactive thyroid gland, Parkinson's disease, side effects to medications, too much caffeine, or anxiety. Tremor can also run in families. The tremor should be evaluated by your physician, who may refer you to a neurologist for further investigation. Often an appropriate medication produces significant relief.

New Drug for Parkinson's

Q. *I've been taking Sinemet and Parlodel for two years to treat Parkinson's disease. I've heard deprenyl is a promising new drug. Is that right?*

A. Deprenyl *(Eldepryl)*, also known as selegiline, does show promise and is being widely used.

Parkinson's disease, a neurological disorder that stiffens muscles, is caused by loss of brain cells that supply dopamine. That chemical transmits nerve signals in parts of the brain that control the muscles.

L-dopa with carbidopa *(Sinemet)* increases dopamine levels in the brain, while bromocriptine *(Parlodel)* increases dopamine's action. Deprenyl, on the other hand, may slow the loss of those brain cells and therefore delay or reduce the need for the other drugs.

Sciatica and Numb Toes

Q. *Last year I had sciatica from my back down to my right leg. The pain cleared up but left me with a kind of numbness in three toes (big toe and adjacent two) that I can't seem to shake. What can I do about this?*

A. Your numbness probably stems from some chronic irritation of the sciatic nerve root as it leaves the spinal cord. This may be caused by a herniated, or "slipped," disk, a disk fragment, or a bone spur. Unfortunately, the longer the numbness lasts, the less likely it is to disappear. A consultation with a neurologist would be advisable.

Sizing Up Seizure Drugs

Q. Our 2½-year-old son has been taking phenobarbital to control his epileptic seizures, but it makes him hyperactive. His doctor suggests switching to Dilantin or Tegretol. Which would be safer, given that he's so young and may be on medication the rest of his life?

A. Both drugs are effective, but carbamazepine (*Tegretol*) may be safer for very long-term use. Both require close monitoring by a physician for possible adverse effects.

Carbamazepine's most common side effects tend to come on early in the course of treatment and are often temporary. Drowsiness and dizziness, for example, usually disappear with time. But allergic skin rashes, sometimes severe, require that the drug be discontinued. The risk of aplastic anemia, in which blood-cell production by the bone marrow is drastically reduced, has slowed acceptance of carbamazepine. Recent evidence, however, suggests that this reaction is extremely rare.

Phenytoin (*Dilantin*) has many side effects when used over the long term. The most common are gum overgrowth and growth of fine hairs on the back and shoulders. Other side effects include interference with the production of vitamin D and, occasionally, development of anemia. Cognitive defects, such as short-term memory impairment, have occurred in adults and require further study in children.

Slapping Gait

Q. What are the cause and treatment of "slap foot," which makes the front of the foot slap down noisily when walking?

A. Slap foot, or what doctors call a slapping gait, results when something goes wrong with the nerves controlling the muscles in front of the lower leg. The weakened muscles can't lift the forefoot, which hits the ground before the heel. The problem could be caused by a bulging or herniated intervertebral disk or a bone spur pressing on the spinal cord. It could also be caused by a damaged or inflamed nerve supplying the front part of the leg. Treatment depends on locating the cause. If no treatment is effective, a brace can be helpful.

Treating a Tremor

Q. *Are there any vitamins, minerals, or specific foods that might help the condition known as "benign essential tremor"?*

A. The medical term "essential" is often applied to conditions for which the cause is not known, and that unfortunately is the case with this troublesome neurological ailment. It sometimes runs in families, so there may be a genetic component. Unfortunately, there is no evidence that any nutritional therapy will improve this trembling of the hands, face, or voice. Small quantities of alcohol may temporarily suppress it, and beta-blocker drugs (such as propranolol or nadolol) frequently help. A recent study with a small number of patients found about half responded well to a drug called methazolamide *(Neptazane)*, also used for glaucoma. However, these medications help the tremor only as long as they're being used. It may be more helpful to minimize intake of substances that can worsen tremors, such as caffeine, certain drugs for asthma, and oral decongestants.

Nose, Mouth, and Throat Disorders

Home Remedies for Canker Sores

Q. *For years I've used a remedy for canker sores that you did not mention in your recent report. I cover the sore with alum for a few moments, then rinse. It's somewhat uncomfortable and leaves an unpleasant taste, but the sore stops hurting and clears up. Is there some reason I should stop using alum?*

A. If it works for you, there's no reason to stop now. From the letters we've received, it seems that everyone has a favorite home remedy for canker sores—alum, baking soda, gentian violet, I-lysine, and others. Although scientific evidence of their efficacy is lacking, these remedies are probably safe when used in such a limited way.

Loss of Taste and Smell

Q. *At the age of 54, I seem to be losing my sense of taste and smell. What might be causing this?*

A. Like hearing and vision, taste and smell tend to deteriorate with age. In addition, various illnesses and injuries can damage the nerves connecting the sense organs to the brain. Loss of smell, for example, can be caused by nasal or sinus infections, nasal polyps, meningitis, or brain tumors. Loss of smell can affect taste. So can allergies, tongue injuries, stroke, or tumors. You should consult your physician to rule out possible underlying disorders.

Sensory Shutdown

Q. *My sense of smell has gradually deteriorated to the point that even pungent odors such as skunk spray don't register. I'm 35 years old and in excellent health with the exception of asthma, for which I take allergy injections, a steroid nasal spray, and other medications. Why am I losing my sense of smell?*

A. Two factors may be to blame. Your nasal passages may be sufficiently swollen from allergy-related causes, including nasal polyps, to limit your ability to detect odors. In addition, long-term use of a nasal spray could affect the smell receptors in your nasal membranes. A consultation with an otorhinolaryngologist (ear, nose, and throat specialist) may be of help.

Bad Taste

Q. *I often notice a metallic taste in my mouth. What causes this and what can I do about it?*

A. Possible causes of your "dysgeusia" or distorted taste, range from allergies and nasal polyps to a prior head trauma or exposure to chemicals. It can also be a side effect of certain medications, particularly the antibiotics metronidazole *(Flagyl)*, clarithromycin *(Biaxin)*, or tetracycline. Sometimes metal fillings in your teeth may be the reason. Most often, however, no cause can be found. In that case, there's nothing to do but wait it out. The sensation may last for years before it mysteriously disappears.

Nay to Nose Surgery?

Q. *How necessary is surgery for a deviated septum? I believe this common operation corrects a birth defect and question its value on my 56-year-old nose.*

A. Most people are born with a straight septum, the cartilage-and-bone partition inside the nose. While some septal deviations are hereditary, many people incur slight deviations from minor childhood mishaps.

Frequently, nasal congestion blamed on a deviated septum is caused by allergies, air pollution, pregnancy, or certain drugs. Short-term use of decongestants can usually clear the blocked airways. (Pregnant women should check with their physician about specific products.)

When the deviation is severe and causes chronic breathing difficulty, repeated sinus infections, or chronic postnasal drip, removal of the obstructing portion of the septum can often provide permanent relief. However, a decision for surgery may be based on inadequate evidence of airway obstruction. So a second opinion should always be sought.

Problems with Nasal Polyps

Q. *I have a nasal polyp that flares up each year for about a month and causes unbearable headaches. I had one removed surgically three years ago, but now the problem has recurred. Steroid nasal sprays seem to help, but I'm worried about using them. Are there any safer treatments?*

A. It's probably safe to continue with the sprays, especially for just one month a year. Very little of the steroid gets absorbed into the blood. A nasal polyp is actually swollen sinus tissue that protrudes into the nasal cavity. Polyps occur singly or in grapelike clusters. Since they're often caused by allergies, polyps can be treated the way allergies are—with antihistamines, decongestants, corticosteroid sprays, or even allergy shots. Alternatively, polyps can be removed surgically under local anesthesia. But as you can attest, additional ones can eventually appear.

Recurrent Sinus Infections

Q. *What can I do about recurrent sinus infections? They clear up temporarily after antibiotics, but return in a couple of months. My doctor says X rays show thickening in my sinuses.*

A. That thickening is due to chronic inflammation of the sinus lining. And an inflamed lining secretes excessive amounts of mucus, which predisposes you to yet another infection. You may need aggressive treatment with longer courses of antibiotics to break the cycle. Failing that, you should be evaluated by an otorhinolaryngologist (ear, nose, and throat specialist) for possible surgery to permit better drainage.

Postnasal Drip

Q. *I suffer from postnasal drip, which constantly fills my throat with phlegm. What can I do about it?*

A. Probably not much. Postnasal drip is typically caused by air pollution, allergies, or infections. The irritated membranes in your nose and sinuses thicken and produce too much mucus. When the condition becomes chronic, it's often difficult to tell what caused it. And it's seldom cured.

Side effects from the standard medications used for postnasal drip—antibiotics, antihistamines, and decongestants—often outweigh their meager benefits. (Decongestants can also lead to dependency.) If you should try these drugs and they don't work, see an otorhinolaryngologist (ear, nose, and throat specialist). Once cysts, polyps, and tumors have been ruled out, either a corticosteroid nasal spray or cortisone injections into the nasal membranes may help.

Nosebleeds

Q. *I've had allergies since I was a child. Four years ago, I had an operation for a broken nose. Now my nose bleeds if I happen to rub it— even only gently. Why?*

A. The problem probably has nothing to do with your broken nose or operation. But it may be related to your allergies—or, more precisely, your allergy medications. Antihistamines and decongestants can dry the mucous lining of the nasal passages. Rubbing, scratching, or other trauma can easily cause bleeding in a dry nose. To lessen drying, minimize your use of those medications and keep your environment comfortably humidified.

Noninhaled Tobacco

Q. *Health reports often warn about the dangers of cigarette smoking. What are the risks of tobacco that's not inhaled, such as that of pipes, cigars, and chewing tobacco?*

A. The fact is that some pipe and cigar smokers do inhale, even unconsciously. Aside from the known risks of inhaled smoke, the main danger is cancer of the mouth and throat. The risk is greater in people who also drink a lot of alcohol. In addition, nicotine is easily absorbed through the lining of the mouth, which increases the risk of coronary heart disease.

Pharyngitis Demystified

Q. *I've seen references to "pharyngitis" and haven't been able to figure out what it is. My dictionary says it's inflammation of the pharynx, which is "the part of the vertebrate alimentary canal between the cavity of the mouth and the esophagus." Please translate.*

A. It's a sore throat.

Thrush

Q. *A few months ago I developed "thrush"—whitish patches on my tongue and on the back of my throat—after a six-day course of intravenous antibiotics. Apparently, the antibiotics killed the normal protective bacteria in my mouth, allowing the thrush to develop. Now I'm concerned about my intestinal bacteria as well. So I've been taking L. acidophilus and bifidus supplements to reestablish those bacteria. Is that the right thing to do?*

A. No. The bacterial imbalance that follows use of antibiotics may indeed allow other bacteria or fungi to take hold. These include the candida that cause thrush. But the "intestinal flora" supplements you mention have never been shown to help prevent or treat that imbalance.

You should treat the candida with an effective antifungal medicine, such as oral nystatin (*Mycostatin*). The usual bacterial population will return to your mouth and intestinal tract on its own.

Aging: Hard to Swallow?

Q. *Older people often seem to choke on food, cough a lot while eating, or swallow "the wrong way." What are the cause and treatment for these reflexes?*

A. As people age, the muscles in the back of the throat and upper esophagus, which are responsible for swallowing, often become less well coordinated. Most older people don't notice this gradual change unless it's compounded by other factors—for instance, poor chewing due to problems with teeth or dentures, or eating or drinking too rapidly.

To help prevent choking, try to chew food well, swallow carefully, and eat in an upright position. If you wear dentures, make sure they fit properly.

Hard to Swallow

Q. *I have esophageal achalasia, which makes swallowing extremely difficult. Other than eating finely chopped food or chewing food thoroughly, is surgery the only way to correct my problem?*

A. No. Only about one out of four patients eventually requires surgery. In achalasia, the muscular ring, or sphincter, between the esophagus and the stomach fails to open adequately when you swallow. Treatment depends on the severity of the condition, which is determined by taking X rays and examining the esophagus through an endoscope, a flexible lighted tube. (Since achalasia may increase the risk of esophageal cancer, endoscopy checks for that possibility as well.)

There are two nonsurgical alternatives. Medications such as nifedipine *(Procardia)* may relax the sphincter. If not, a special instrument can be passed down the throat to widen the sphincter by splitting the constricting muscle fibers.

Rash in the Mouth

Q. *A dermatologist told me that I have lichen planus inside my mouth. Can you tell me more about it?*

A. Lichen planus is a common skin disease that usually appears as small, shiny, extremely itchy, raised pink spots. The condition most often affects the wrists, forearms, or lower legs, but it can also show up on the inside lining of the cheeks as a network of white spots. The cause of lichen planus is unknown.

Physicians typically prescribe a special corticosteroid paste *(Orabase* HCA) to treat lichen planus in the mouth; the skin rash is treated with similar creams. In severe cases, those treatments may be supplemented by corticosteroid injections. Even with treatment, however, the condition can linger for as long as a year and a half, and it may recur.

Coated Tongue

Q. *Recently I noticed a white film on my tongue that I can't seem to remove by brushing. Any suggestions?*

A. First, try to track down the cause of your coated tongue. Sometimes it's a change in diet. If so, try eliminating the suspected offender, and see if the coating disappears. Ask your physician whether the culprit could be a yeast infection or medication you have taken—particularly antibiotics and medications that dry the mouth, such as antihistamines.

When the cause can't be determined or corrected, brushing the tongue with a soft-bristle toothbrush does help some people. Since that didn't help you, you might simply try drinking more fluids. In time, the condition will probably disappear on its own.

Eat and Run

Q. *Why does my nose run while eating or after I eat? It happens with all types of foods, and mainly after dinner.*

A. You're experiencing what's called prandial rhinorrhea, meaning—sure enough—the free discharge of a thin nasal mucus, associated with a meal. Eating activates the autonomic nervous system, which releases the chemical acetylcholine. That in turn gets the body's juices flowing, including saliva and stomach acid as well as nasal mucus and sometimes tears. The degree of reaction varies widely. Usually, the spicier the meal, the greater the reaction.

If your problem is severe, try taking an antihistamine or a decongestant before you eat. If that doesn't do the trick, consult your physician.

☐ OFFICE VISIT
Snoring Can Be Hazardous to Your Health

"I've been suspended. They won't let me drive anymore."

My patient, an obese 38-year-old taxicab driver, said he'd fallen asleep behind the wheel three times in the past five weeks. He'd caused a tie-up at a traffic light, a fire in his front seat (where he'd dropped a lit cigarette), and a collision that demolished the front of his cab.

"I just can't stay awake, and it's getting worse," he said. "My wife's ready to leave me. She's already sleeping in the guest room."

"Why is that?" I asked.

"She can't stand my snoring."

This twist didn't surprise me much. Heavy snoring has indeed driven bedmates from the bedroom. But the popular notion that snoring afflicts everyone except the snorer is false. Snoring may signal an ominous disorder that can cause daytime drowsiness and night-time death.

A Chorus of Snorers

The likelihood of snoring increases with age: In their early thirties, about 20 percent of men and 5 percent of women snore. By age 60, 60 percent of men and 40 percent of women are snoring away.

People snore when the airway narrows where the mouth meets the throat. The inhaled air rushing through the constricted space rattles the soft tissues, creating a raspy sound.

Probably the main cause of snoring is poor muscle tone in that part of the airway, which has no rigid support. When the snorer inhales, the flaccid tissues get sucked inward, partially obstructing the airway. Alcohol, sleeping pills, and tranquilizers encourage snoring by further relaxing those muscles. And when congestion (from a cold or allergy) or deformity (such as a deviated septum) blocks the nasal passages, breathing exerts even greater pressure on the airway.

Snorers usually have a narrower airway to begin with. Nearly all snorers have an elongated soft palate (the rear part of the roof of the mouth) or uvula (the triangular flap hanging down in the back of the throat). Obese people are more likely than others to snore, possibly because they have bulky airway tissues. Smoking cigarettes can irritate those soft tissues, making them swell. Rarely, the airway is narrowed by a cyst or tumor.

An Alarming Lull

If the airway is completely blocked, the din suddenly—and ominously—ceases. The sleeper has stopped breathing. Anywhere from a few seconds to half a minute later, the buildup of carbon dioxide in the blood rouses the sleeper, who snorts, gasps for breath, and almost immediately resumes sleeping. These episodes are seldom recalled the next day. About 2.5 million Americans, most of them obese, experience such nighttime breathing lapses, known as sleep apnea.

The cycle of snoring, apnea, arousal, and sleep may repeat hundreds of times a night. The snorer gets little or no deep sleep and thus may be extremely drowsy the next day. The periodic lack of oxygen may contribute to cardiovascular problems, including high blood pressure and coronary heart disease. Most important, the breathing problems can produce irregular heart rhythms, which can lead to sudden death.

Self-Help for Snorers

If you snore lightly or occasionally, these steps may help:

□ Lose weight.
□ Stop smoking.
□ Avoid alcohol, sleeping pills, and tranquilizers at bedtime.
□ Sleep on your side. (When you're on your back, your tongue and soft palate tend to slip back into the airway.) A tennis ball sewn into the back of your pajama top may force you to roll over.
□ Don't sleep with your neck bent forward, which narrows the airway. Avoid thick pillows.
□ Use nasal decongestants for colds and allergies.

More than 300 antisnoring gadgets have been patented. These include collars or straps for the chin, head, or neck; tongue retainers; and electric gizmos that zap you when you snore. For most people, the only way these contraptions prevent snoring is by preventing sleep.

Treating the Serious Snorer

If you snore heavily, you should talk to your physician. It may be a sign of sleep apnea. Not long ago, the only treatment for sleep apnea was tracheostomy (cutting a breathing hole in the neck below the Adam's apple). Newer treatments have almost entirely supplanted that procedure. There are now two main options:

1. *Continuous positive airway pressure.* A pump attached to a nose mask forces air into the upper airway to keep it from collapsing. The device is effective, provided you can sleep with a mask clamped to your face.
2. *Surgery.* The airway can be widened by cutting out the uvula and part of the soft palate, or tightening the relaxed tissues at the back of the throat. This operation eliminates snoring in most patients and apnea in about half. Surgery can also remove the rare cyst or growth, or correct nasal deformities.

Snoring Silenced

I spoke with my patient's wife, who described his snorting and gasping. That confirmed my suspicions of sleep apnea. I referred him to a sleep disorders clinic, where sleep monitoring revealed a potentially lethal cardiac rhythm disturbance. Medication was prescribed to prevent that arrhythmia. After evaluation by a throat specialist, the cab driver had his airway surgically widened, quit smoking, and started to lose weight. He returned to his cab, and his wife rejoined him in their now-quiet bedroom.

Pain Medications

Aspirin for Chicken Pox?

Q. *I've heard that you shouldn't give aspirin to children who have chicken pox, but what about adults?*

A. For adults, there's no risk in taking aspirin to relieve the pain and itch of chicken pox. However, children under the age of 16 who have chicken pox, flu, or even an ordinary upper-respiratory infection must not be given aspirin. It can trigger Reye's syndrome, a rare but often fatal childhood disease. Safe alternatives to aspirin include acetaminophen (*Tylenol*) and ibuprofen (*Advil, Nuprin*).

Aspirin, Ibuprofen, and Clotting

Q. *Is there any difference between aspirin and ibuprofen in their tendency to inhibit the blood-clotting action of platelets?*

A. Yes—though it's a difference in degree. A daily dose of three 200-milligram ibuprofen tablets (*Advil, Nuprin*) can inhibit platelet function for about 24 hours. It takes only about one-third of a single 325-milligram aspirin tablet to inhibit platelets for up to a week. While people with bleeding disorders must avoid aspirin, they may be able to use ibuprofen under a doctor's supervision.

Aspirin and Hearing

Q. *I frequently take aspirin and have lately begun to wonder if it affects my hearing. Can it?*

A. Yes. Hearing loss and tinnitus (ringing in the ears) have been recognized for more than a century as signs of aspirin toxicity. When those problems are caused by too much aspirin, both problems disappear on reducing the aspirin dosage. If either problem persists, check with your physician.

Aspirin Gone Bad

Q. I have always heard that you should discard aspirin when it begins to smell like vinegar. The last bottle I bought has an expiration date of two years from now, but it already has that vinegary odor. Is such aspirin harmful?

A. No, just less effective. The odor indicates that the drug is breaking down into its constituent parts. That happens gradually, but begins as soon as you first open the bottle. Even fresh aspirin has some vinegary smell. But if the odor is very strong in a previously unopened bottle, replace it. To slow the decomposition, store aspirin in a cool, dry place (not the bathroom) and keep the cap tightly closed.

How to Take Aspirin

Q. I've been taking aspirin regularly every other day because of its apparent ability to prevent heart attacks. What is the best way to take it?

A. To lessen the chance of stomach irritation, aspirin should be taken with or after meals. Wash it down with an 8-ounce glass of water.

The contents of your stomach can back up into the esophagus when you recline. Any undissolved aspirin can therefore irritate the esophagus. So, to prevent heartburn, avoid lying down for 15 to 30 minutes after taking the aspirin.

Pain in the Neck

Q. *When I walk uphill rapidly, I get a slight pain in the left side of my neck. My doctor ordered a treadmill test, which showed nothing abnormal. I'm 60 years old. What could the pain be?*

A. There are two main possibilities: One is simple arthritic or muscular pain. If holding your head in certain positions sparks the pain, the problem might well be musculoskeletal.

Or it could be an atypical form of angina pectoris, a symptom of insufficient blood circulation to the heart. The pain is usually centered in the chest but may sometimes be felt only in the neck.

If physical exertion triggers the pain, coronary heart disease must be suspected. That's why your doctor tested you on a treadmill—to see whether the exercise would either provoke the pain or reveal evidence of inadequate circulation on an electrocardiogram.

Unfortunately, a normal result on a standard treadmill stress test does not necessarily exclude coronary disease. To rule that out more definitively, you may need a nuclear stress test, in which a radioactive chemical is injected into the bloodstream during exercise and the heart is scanned by a radiation detector. If the nuclear test shows an abnormality, then angiography *may* be necessary.

Pain-Relief Dilemma

Q. *Since the painkiller Percocet contains acetaminophen, I wonder if it's safe for prolonged use. The label on acetaminophen warns against taking it longer than 10 days, and I've read that excessive use can cause liver damage. What can you tell me about this?*

A. Irreversible liver damage can result from even a single large overdose of acetaminophen—meaning more than 10 grams (about 30 regular-strength tablets). At normal dosages, prolonged use of acetaminophen won't harm the liver in most people. But heavy drinkers or people with existing liver damage should avoid the drug.

Long-term, daily use of acetaminophen may also increase the risk of kidney damage. So anyone taking it regularly should have a periodic blood test for kidney function. Taking *Percocet*, in particular, requires an extra note of caution. That combination product also contains an opium-derived narcotic and, taken for a long time or in large doses, it can be habit-forming. Extended use is best limited to cases of severe chronic pain and should be monitored by a physician.

Trigeminal Neuralgia

Q. *I have trigeminal neuralgia, which causes excruciating pain on one side of my face. The drug* Tegretol *eliminates the pain but leaves me confused, drowsy, and depressed. Is there any alternative treatment?*

A. To start with, your physician may be able to reduce your dosage of carbamazepine (*Tegretol*) without compromising the drug's effectiveness. If that doesn't work, your physician might try other drugs, such as phenytoin (*Dilantin*) or amitriptyline (*Elavil*).

It's also possible to deaden the particular nerve that's causing the pain, using alcohol or glycerol injections, nerve blocks, radio frequency waves through the skin, or surgery. However, those procedures can leave part of your face permanently numb.

Wary of *Darvocet-N*

Q. *I have intermittent claudication. When the pain keeps me awake at night or is too much to ignore, I take Darvocet-N, usually two to three tablets a day. The package insert warns not to exceed six tablets a day. Given my daily intake, is Darvocet-N dangerous?*

A. Your symptoms suggest that you may benefit from further medical evaluation. Intermittent claudication, an aching or cramp-like pain in the calves arising from poor blood supply to the legs, typically occurs during walking and subsides promptly with rest. Discomfort that persists may reflect more serious vascular disease that requires treatment.

As for *Darvocet-N*: One of this drug's active ingredients is acetaminophen, a painkiller preferred by many people who experience stomach irritation with aspirin. However, a recent study found that long-term, daily use of acetaminophen may increase the risk of kidney or liver damage. When long-term use is unavoidable, have your kidney function monitored by a periodic blood test.

Feldene Side Effects

Q. *I have a gnawing ache in my left thigh, diagnosed as pressure on a nerve from a bulging vertebral disk. My doctor prescribed* Feldene, *which helps. But will I have trouble with side effects if I keep using it?*

A. Perhaps. About 20 percent of patients who take piroxicam (*Feldene*) report adverse effects—most often gastrointestinal complaints, such as upset stomach, nausea, constipation, diarrhea, or flatulence. Such problems force about 5 percent of users to stop taking the drug.

Like aspirin, piroxicam and all other Nonsteroidal anti-inflammatory drugs (such as fenoprofen, ibuprofen, and naproxen) can cause slight blood loss in the stool, although it may not be readily visible. Over a period of months, this can cause anemia. Your physician should check your blood count every two or three months. People who bleed easily, take anticoagulants, or are sensitive to aspirin should avoid piroxicam.

☐ Respiratory Infections

Antibiotics for a Bad Cold

Q. *I've had two particularly bad colds over the past year. Both times, my doctor prescribed antibiotics. I thought that a cold is a viral infection and that antibiotics aren't effective against viruses. Why the antibiotics?*

A. That depends. Antibiotics indeed won't do anything for a viral infection such as the common cold. But sometimes a cold virus leads to a bacterial infection in the sinus or bronchial airways, which does require antibiotics.

A physician typically makes that decision by looking for signs of bacterial infection. Sinus infections can produce a thick, yellow discharge from the nose, tenderness or pain just above or below the eyes, and perhaps a slight fever. Bronchial infections can also cause fever as well as a cough that brings up greenish yellow sputum or even some blood.

If you have none of those symptoms, you probably shouldn't take antibiotics. The drugs can cause such side effects as nausea, diarrhea, and rashes. They can also kill off the body's own protective bacteria, allowing fungal infections to grow in the mouth, intestines, or vagina.

Contagious Colds

Q. *My friend says a cold is no longer contagious once you start having symptoms—sneezing, dripping, and so on.*

A. Quite the contrary. Colds spread easily through contact with those nasal secretions. When the secretions dry up, *then* you're no longer contagious.

Where There's Smoke

Q. *A year or so ago I was diagnosed as having a bronchial infection caused by Hemophilus influenza bacteria. Despite having taken three or four antibiotics, I still have a very productive cough. Could the fact that I smoke cigarettes be hampering my recovery?*

A. Very likely. Not only do smokers experience more respiratory infections than nonsmokers do, but they also are likely to have more difficulty recovering. Smoking destroys cilia, the tiny filaments that help to move infected mucus up and out of the lungs. And the ability of the lungs to repair tissue damage is impaired by years of smoking. It shouldn't surprise you to learn that the best solution is to quit.

Skin Care

Scratching an Itch

Q. *For months I've been suffering from an annoying itch. It starts in one spot, I scratch it, and it turns red and bumpy. Then it disappears and starts up again somewhere else. I've been taking* Seldane, *which helps, but I'm worried. What's wrong with me?*

A. The red, bumpy rashes you describe are probably the result of scratching, not the cause of the itch. Unexplained generalized itching, called pruritis, has several possible causes. Older people often itch in the winter because their skin becomes drier. Using water-soluble lubricating oils, bathing less frequently, and running a room humidifier may help. Certain systemic diseases, such as diabetes, liver disease, and some forms of cancer can also cause itching. These can easily be excluded by appropriate tests. If the cause is unknown, antihistamines, such as hydroxyzine (*Atarax*) and terfenadine (*Seldane*) can help.

Note: The FDA has warned against the use of terfenadine together with the antifungal drug ketoconazole (*Nizoral*) or the antibiotic erythromycin. Interaction with these drugs can boost blood levels of terfenadine to the danger point, risking potentially fatal heart rhythm abnormalities. Astemizole (*Hismanal*), an antihistamine, interacts similarly and also should not be used together with ketoconazole or erythromycin.

Itching All Over

Q. *For the past two years, I've itched from my scalp to the soles of my feet, including the palms of my hands, my ears, and my eyes. There is no rash. At night the itching is accompanied by muscular spasms in my legs and a burning sensation. Please help.*

A. Persistent itching can be caused by allergies to food or medications, and by skin disorders such as scabies (which don't always have visible signs). The burning sensation you've experienced could be a sign of nerve inflammation. A physical exam is needed to find the cause for your itching. If your physician can find no treatable cause, he or she may recommend an oral antihistamine such as hydroxyzine (*Atarax, Vistaril*) to relieve the symptoms.

Eczema

Q. *I have eczema on my hands and feet—blisters, itching, peeling, cracking, and bleeding—that gets worse in the winter. What can I do about it?*

A. Since scratching the skin prolongs the problem, avoid any irritant, such as wool, synthetic fibers, animal fur, or soap. Any of them might set off the itch-scratch cycle. To soothe your skin, keep it well lubricated with bland lotions. Over-the-counter hydrocortisone creams (*Caldecort, Cortaid*) may also help, but when used over a long period of time, they can thin the skin. This can reduce the skin's effectiveness as a protective barrier and make it more vulnerable to trauma. Avoid preparations that contain anesthetics, antihistamines, or other chemicals alleged to relieve itching; they may cause allergic reactions when applied to inflamed skin.

Poison Ivy Protection?

Q. *I'm allergic to poison ivy and periodically break out with itching and blisters. Are there drugs or shots I can take to prevent a recurrence?*

A. Unfortunately not. The rash caused by poison ivy is a type of allergic contact dermatitis, a reaction to a potent chemical in the plant. Efforts to desensitize people to poison ivy, using injections or pills containing small amounts of the chemical, have generally been unsuccessful. The best protection is to steer clear of the plant or to wear gloves and other protective clothing when gardening or tramping through the woods. Then, make sure to wash those gloves and other protective clothing if you have reason to suspect they might have touched a poison ivy plant.

Scabies and Itching

Q. *You mention dry skin and a few systemic diseases as possible causes of unexplained itching. Doesn't scabies also cause itching?*

A. Yes, it does. Scabies is a very itchy skin disorder caused by a tiny mite. Usually passed directly from one person to another, the insect can also be transmitted by contaminated clothing or bedding. Scabies is most common in children but can also affect adults. The prescription drug lindane (*Kwell*), applied as a cream or a lotion for up to 24 hours, generally kills the mites and cures scabies. (Read the label warnings carefully.) The itch can take weeks to subside even after the disease has been successfully treated.

Harried by Hives

Q. *About a week ago I suddenly developed hives—blistery blotches on my skin that seem to appear and disappear within a short time. Why would hives wait until I was 67 years old before appearing? What could be causing them?*

A. Hives can show up at any age. Unfortunately, their cause remains a mystery close to 70 percent of the time. Allergies to food, food additives, medication, or other ingested substances probably account for most cases. If the hives recur frequently, keeping a diary of your food and medication might provide a clue to the specific agent. Cold, heat, and even physical pressure can give some people hives as well.

Anxiety and emotional upset are overrated as a cause of hives but can provoke an occasional outbreak. While you're searching for an explanation for your case, antihistamines can relieve the discomfort. Occasionally, temporary use of a prescription steroid medication may be necessary.

Dry-Lip Distress

Q. *I am troubled by very dry lips for which no cause has been found. Following my doctor's advice, I use cortisone cream and special lipsticks, but the condition persists. I have also tried all kinds of vitamins, to no avail. Any further advice?*

A. Extremely dry lips, known as cheilitis, can sometimes be traced to a contact allergy (to lipsticks, lip salves, mouthwash, or toothpaste), to nighttime drooling or frequent lip licking, or, rarely, to a deficiency of iron or vitamin B_2 (riboflavin). Often, however, the cause remains obscure. Systematically avoiding each suspect product—one at a time—may uncover the one responsible. With toothpaste, for example, try switching brands. Also steer clear of oral medications containing antihistamines, which tend to dry the mucous membranes of the mouth. To moisten and protect your lips, use a nonirritating product such as petroleum jelly *(Vaseline)*, and apply a lip balm containing a sunblock when outdoors.

Shingles: The Aftereffects

Q. *About a year ago, my wife contracted a severe case of shingles. Although the rash is gone now, the severe pain persists. Her doctors have prescribed only pain-relief pills. Is there a permanent cure?*

A. The pain that remains after an attack of shingles is known as postherpetic neuralgia, and it is notoriously hard to vanquish.

Some drugs have proven helpful, but not for all people. These include capsaicin (often sold as *Zostrix*), a topical medication; amitriptyline *(Elavil)*, an antidepressant; phenytoin *(Dilantin)* and carbamazepine *(Tegretol)*, both anticonvulsants; and injections of corticosteroids. In other people, only time brings relief; the pain can last for months or years.

Some dermatologists now prescribe oral cortisone, taken for three weeks after shingles first appears, to prevent the pain that persists after an attack. But the efficacy of this treatment is unproven.

A Large, Red Nose

Q. *I have a friend whose nose is quite large and very red. He takes an antibiotic for the problem. What causes this?*

A. Your friend probably has rosacea (also called acne rosacea and adult acne), a chronic skin disease that causes a reddish/bluish rash over the cheeks and nose. (It is often associated with swelling.) Rosacea is most common in middle age, especially among women. Although the cause remains a mystery, the disease can be successfully controlled with oral tetracyclines or topical antibiotics such as metronidazole *(MetroGel)*.

Rosacea

Q. *I have rosacea, mostly on my cheeks. What can I do about it?*

A. In some people, avoiding hot or spicy foods, hot beverages, and alcohol will minimize this chronic blood-vessel inflammation, which appears as redness or pustules on the cheeks, nose, chin, forehead, or eyelids. If those measures don't help, your physician can prescribe oral or topical antibiotics that will control the condition, just as they control acne. But avoid hydrocortisone cream; long-term use can cause changes that resemble rosacea itself.

Stubborn Rosacea

Q. *I've been taking antibiotics for rosacea, but after three months the results are disappointing. Is there another treatment option?*

A. Rosacea—a chronic skin disorder that produces redness or pustules on the cheeks, nose, chin, forehead, or eyelids—tends to be a persistent problem. If antibiotics don't do the trick, your physician might prescribe the acne medication isotretinoin (*Accutane*), which can often clear up a particularly stubborn case. But even that can take more than six months to be effective.

Skin Growths

Q. *I have a bad case of seborrheic keratoses—grayish, molelike growths all over my torso. They're not painful, but they are unsightly. What should I do?*

A. Seborrheic keratoses don't become cancerous, so they're purely a cosmetic matter. A dermatologist could remove them easily, since the soft growths don't adhere strongly to the skin. Most dermatologists simply freeze the skin to numb it and then scrape the growths off with a curette (a rounded cutting instrument). If necessary, an electric current first destroys the growths.

The procedure produces minimal bleeding and the wounds heal without scarring. However, you may be uncomfortable while you're healing, and it could cost several hundred dollars to have the more pervasive growths removed.

A Formidable Fungus

Q. *I've had athlete's foot for more than 10 years and have been using prescription creams such as Loprox and Lotrimin to keep it under control. It's a very stubborn fungus, in part because it has gone under one* *of my toenails. Is it okay to continue using these medications regularly? Can you offer an alternative?*

A. It's safe to continue with the creams you mention. You should also maintain good foot hygiene: Dry between toes after bathing, rub away dead skin, and apply an antifungal powder for daytime use. An alternative would be the oral antifungal medication ketoconazole (*Nizoral*), a potent drug generally used only for major fungal infections. A preferable oral alternative would be griseofulvin (*Fulvicin, Grifulvin, Grisactin*). This prescription drug is reasonably safe, although it can increase sensitivity to sunlight. Liver function and blood counts also need to be monitored periodically. Expect to continue the therapy for at least a year. Even if the fungus completely clears, there's a high probability of recurrence. Overall, you're probably better off continuing to use whatever topical measures have helped you in the past.

Antifungal Medication

Q. *I have had a fungal infection of the toenail for many years and have tried various topical treatments. My podiatrist recommends trying Nizoral for about six months. What are the risks of taking this drug? I can't take griseofulvin.*

A. Ketoconazole (*Nizoral*) is a potent drug that is generally reserved for major fungal infections, since it can cause liver damage and other serious side effects. This drug, taken orally, should not be used for a fungal toenail infection, which is essentially a cosmetic problem—especially since drug treatment to eradicate such an infection must continue for at least a year. Griseofulvin (*Fulvicin, Grifulvin, Grisactin*), the only other oral drug treatment for fungal toenail infections, is more benign, but can also cause side effects including headache and stomach pain. Since you are unable to take this drug, your other options are to have the nail removed by a surgeon or podiatrist—or continue living with it as you have in the past.

Toenail Fungus

Q. My toenail has a fungal infection. I've seen two dermatologists, who prescribed three drugs, Loprox, Mycelex, and Spectazole. After a year and a half, the condition hasn't improved. Are there any other treatments?

A. Yes, but the risks and costs may not be worth the benefit. The antifungal medications griseofulvin (Fulvicin, Grifulvin, Grisactin) and ketoconazole (Nizoral), both taken orally, do reach the infection. But while they keep fungus from spreading to new nail tissue, they don't root it out of tissue that's already infected. So you have to keep taking the drug for at least a year, until the nail grows out completely. Such treatment is expensive and can cause side effects, including allergic reactions, headaches, and stomach distress. And oral ketoconazole is a potent drug that can cause liver damage. As a last resort, you could undergo surgery to permanently remove the nail.

As for the topical drugs you've been taking, they're useless, since they don't reach the base of the nail under the cuticle. That's where the nail forms and infection breeds.

Since these infections are almost always harmless, it may be best to leave them untreated unless they cause discomfort.

Cracked Heels

Q. Winter or summer, the skin on my heels cracks and splits, sometimes to the point of bleeding. What causes this problem and how can I rid myself of it?

A. First see your physician to check for fungus infection or psoriasis. If those are ruled out, your heels are probably cracking because the skin is too dry. A common treatment involves "moisture trapping"—tap-water baths followed by immediate application of a non-irritating agent such as mineral oil or petroleum jelly before putting on socks and shoes. Other creams and lotions containing water or fragrances may exacerbate the problem, so it's best to avoid them.

Removing Blackheads

Q. *What's the safest, most effective way to remove blackheads on the nose or elsewhere on the face?*

A. If your blackheads are associated with facial acne, seek professional help because of the possibility of infection. For the occasional blackhead, first wash your face (and hands) with soap and warm water, then press down the skin around the blackhead to extrude the oxidized matter plugging the pore. Contrary to myth, this practice will neither enlarge your pores nor leave you with scars.

Tetracycline for Acne

Q. *I've been taking tetracycline for several years to treat my adult acne. Are there any side effects?*

A. Usually only minor ones. Tetracycline and other antibiotics help suppress acne-promoting bacteria in the skin's oil glands. Doctors often prescribe long-term tetracycline treatment for moderately severe acne. After a few weeks at full dosage, the dose is reduced to the smallest amount that will control the problem. Years of experience—thousands of patients and millions of prescriptions—have shown that side effects are usually mild and disappear when the drug is discontinued. Among the most common ones are diarrhea, stomach cramps, and vaginal yeast infections. In some people, tetracycline makes the skin more sensitive to ultraviolet radiation—and more susceptible to severe sunburn. Pregnant or breast-feeding women should avoid tetracycline; it may discolor the teeth of the fetus or newborn infant and slow the growth of the infant's teeth and bones.

If you are taking any other drugs along with tetracycline, you should tell your doctor, since some drugs may decrease the effect of tetracycline. Conversely, if you are taking oral contraceptives containing estrogen along with tetracycline, the tetracycline may decrease the effect of the birth-control pills and thus increase the possibility of unwanted pregnancy.

Acne Scars in Middle Age

Q. *I'm in my early forties. Because of teenage acne, I suffer from a severely pitted and pockmarked complexion. Is there any treatment or surgical procedure that I can undergo to relieve this condition?*

A. A procedure called dermabrasion, in which the skin is literally sanded down, can make scars less obvious and improve overall appearance. This procedure is usually performed under local anesthesia, and can be done by a dermatologist or plastic surgeon on an outpatient basis. After dermabrasion, the skin remains uncomfortably raw for 10 to 14 days; redness may linger for as long as several months.

Cysts on the Scalp

Q. *My brother and I suffer from sebaceous cysts on the scalp. As the cysts enlarge, they itch and hurt when bumped. We've had several of them removed, but they're back in the same places within a few years. Is there any way to get rid of these growths permanently?*

A. When located in the scalp, a skin cyst (properly called a pilar cyst or wen) generally originates with a hair follicle. Elsewhere on the body, a skin cyst (or epidermoid cyst) usually originates with a sebaceous gland duct. Both kinds are benign, saclike swellings beneath the surface of the skin.

Most skin cysts don't need to be removed unless they become infected, painful, or cosmetically unacceptable. If a surgeon removes an entire cyst intact, it won't reform, but more cysts can occur elsewhere. Indeed, many people who tend to form skin cysts have multiple occurrences.

Electrolysis and Moles

Q. *I've been going for electrolysis to remove the hairs that grow from several moles on my face. One dermatologist told me it's dangerous to* *have electrolysis on mole hairs. Another said it's perfectly safe. Who's right?*

A. The one who said it's safe. Some people believe that removing hairs or otherwise disturbing a mole might trigger cancerous changes. However, there's no evidence to support that notion.

Farewell to Keloid Scars

Q. *I've had keloids on my chest for 25 years and they seem to get thicker and more itchy each day. I've had them removed by both conventional and laser surgery and injected with cortisone, but they always come back. Can anything more be done?*

A. Though you've had all available treatments for keloids, you may not have had an aggressive-enough course of postoperative cortisone injections.

Keloids are thick, raised, ropy scars that can occur after a surgical procedure or accidental laceration. The tendency to develop keloids appears to be hereditary. In certain people—particularly blacks and Asians—recurrence is common and hard to avoid.

Consumers Union's plastic surgery consultants advise removing the keloid and immediately injecting the area with cortisone. Additional injections should be given at the first sign of itching, which foreshadows the keloid's reappearance. Within two years, most keloids treated this way are permanently banished. Keloids that aren't bothersome in comfort or appearance can be safely left alone.

No Cure for Vitiligo

Q. *I have had vitiligo for more than 20 years. When I was first diagnosed, I was told there was no treatment for this condition. Is that still the case?*

A. Yes and no. There's still no cure for vitiligo, the patchy loss of skin pigmentation. But newer, more sophisticated skin dyes—

hydroxyacetone, for example—can help to camouflage the whitish patches. Oral medications called psoralens can sometimes sensitize any remaining pigment cells to stimulation by ultraviolet light, helping to retard further loss of skin color. But this treatment may increase the risk of skin cancer and should be reserved for severe cases. Unfortunately, treatment with psoralens usually isn't effective in cases as long-standing as yours. Vitiligo patches can be especially vulnerable to sunburn, so the use of sunscreens is recommended.

Dermatitis from Hair Dye

Q. *Having dyed my hair for the past two years, I am now suffering the consequences—acute dermatitis. According to two dermatologists, the results could have been much worse. What happened?*

A. You seem to have developed a sensitivity to the chemical paraphenylenediamine, a component of many hair dyes. This can cause local swelling and blistering of the scalp. "Cross-sensitization" often occurs, which means that you may now experience a similar reaction to other dyes, certain anesthetics, and even to PABA (the active ingredient in most sunscreens). From now on, you would be wise to use hypoallergenic products whenever they are available.

Purple People

Q. *When I was a marine stationed in the tropics, jock itch was a common problem. The smiling medic would swab on gentian violet, and you'd walk away cured (on fire, but cured). Why didn't you mention that old standby in your article on topical antifungals?*

A. Because few doctors use it anymore. Twenty to 30 years ago, gentian violet (methylrosaniline) was a popular remedy for skin or vaginal problems caused by fungi or bacteria. It was even taken by mouth for intestinal worms. Gentian violet has been replaced by more effective drugs that don't turn you or your socks or underwear purple.

Spotting Skin Cancer

Q. *Should a thorough inspection of the skin be part of a comprehensive physical examination?*

A. Yes. Each year more than 500,000 new cases of skin cancer are diagnosed in the United States, and more than 7,000 people die from the disease. Total body examinations are crucial for early detection and treatment of both skin cancers and premalignant skin lesions. Removal of the lesions usually results in a complete cure, especially if they are detected at an early stage.

If your doctor fails to include a total body exam in your physical, ask for it. If you're at increased risk for skin cancer (because of previous cancerous lesions, family history, or fair complexion), you may want to consult a dermatologist for the exam.

Tanning Lotions and Pills

Q. *Are tanning lotions and tanning pills safe?*

A. Yes and no, respectively. The lotions usually contain dihydroxyacetone, or DHA. They can create an uneven, somewhat off-colored, orangy tan, but they're safe enough.

Tanning pills are not only unsafe, they're illegal. The FDA has approved canthaxanthin, the pills' active ingredient, only for use at very low levels to color some foods and drugs. Used in tanning pills, the dye turns the skin golden orange. It can also build up in the retina and liver, and cause skin reactions, itching, and abnormal liver function tests.

The FDA first warned against the use of such tanning pills in 1981. Since then, the agency has banned the products and seized them occasionally but has not been able to keep them off the market. Bearing such names as *BronzeGlo*, *Darker Tan*, and *Orobronze*, these pills are still marketed through mail-order ads in newspapers and bodybuilding magazines. They're also sold at some health-food stores and tanning salons.

Easy Bruising

Q. *I'm 75 years old and have purpura. What can I do about it?*

A. That depends on the cause. Purpura is a catchall term for bleeding into the skin, which creates purple bruises. Anything that affects the surface blood vessels or platelets (blood cells essential to clotting) can cause purpura. The most likely cause of your purpura is simply the loss, with age, of the protective skin tissue around those blood vessels. There's no treatment for the condition, although avoiding bumps and/or pressure on the skin may help.

However, you should see a physician to rule out more serious problems. These include allergies and other reactions to drugs (including aspirin) and diseases affecting the platelets or bone marrow.

Discoid Lupus

Q. *My husband was recently told he might have discoid lupus, although lab tests were normal. Is this a dangerous disease?*

A. Not by itself. Discoid lupus erythematosus typically causes red, round, scaly rashes. It is, however, related to a more serious disease, systemic lupus erythematosus. Systemic lupus can affect just about every part of the body, including the kidneys and other vital organs.

A skin biopsy can identify discoid lupus; special blood tests are required to identify systemic lupus. Up to 20 percent of patients who have the discoid rash also have the systemic disease. If your husband has discoid lupus but blood tests do not detect systemic lupus, he has about a 95 percent chance of not developing the systemic disease.

A Bathroom Sunburn?

Q. *I use an infrared bulb to warm my bathroom. How much ultraviolet (UV) radiation is given off by these bulbs?*

A. The amount of UV radiation emitted by an infrared bulb is negligible—even less than that emitted by an ordinary bulb.

Split Fingernails

Q. *I'm concerned about my fingernails repeatedly splitting to the quick. What can I take to strenthen them and prevent splits?*

A. Nothing you ingest—including the oft-recommended gelatin and calcium—will strengthen your fingernails. Splitting is most often caused by a minor injury to the nail itself. The biggest culprit is water—more specifically, alternating periods of wetness and dryness. So avoid soaking your hands in water. The overuse of nail polish remover can also cause splitting. Other persistent nail deformities—ridging, pitting, and odd shapes—may reflect chronic diseases or a previous acute illness.

▭ OFFICE VISIT

Scratching an Itch

"Let me tell you, Cassius, you yourself are much condemned to have an itching palm," declared Brutus during a feisty encounter with his coconspirator in Shakespeare's *Julius Caesar*. By indulging his corrupt impulses, Cassius earned the condemnation of his more honorable partner.

In life as in art, scratching a persistent itch, while pleasurable in the moment, can condemn you to greater discomfort in the long run. Far better to get to the root of the itch. There's often an underlying problem that can be corrected.

What Makes You Itch?

The itch sensation travels the same nerve fibers that carry pain signals to the spinal cord and brain. Apparently, scratching brings relief by overwhelming the itch with an even stronger sensation.

When the cause of itching is not obvious, a physician may be tempted to diagnose a "nervous itch." But while emotional stress can aggravate itching, psychological factors are rarely the underlying cause. There's usually a medical explanation.

It's easiest to find the cause when itching is limited to one particular area of the body.

Itching feet or an itch in the groin area is usually due to fungal infection. A mild case may turn the skin reddish brown; in severe cases, the skin can crack, become raw, and even bleed. You can treat a mild infection with over-the-counter antifungal creams and powders, such as clotrimazole *(Lotrimin AF)* or miconazole *(Micatin)*. Severe inflammation could indicate a bacterial infection on top of the fungal infection. In that case, an antifungal product could make the problem worse; see your doctor instead.

Anal itching can also be caused by fungal infections—as well as by hemorrhoids, skin fissures, sweating, worms, or poor anal hygiene. Each problem has its own treatment, ranging from careful cleansing to hydrocortisone cream.

Scabies, which can cause intense itching just about anywhere on the body, is caused by a microscopic mite that burrows under the skin. If you look closely, you'll see little ridges or dotted lines ending in tiny blisters. Treatment consists of using a pesticide-containing cream or lotion. Even after the mite has been successfully eradicated, though, the itch can persist for weeks.

When Scratching Hurts

Sometimes, localized itching can actually be caused by scratching. This condition, known as neurodermatitis, is not an actual nerve disorder but rather a vicious spiral of itching and repeated scratching that leads to gradual thickening and darkening of the skin; the area then itches more than ever. Neurodermatitis is seen most often on the nape or side of the neck, but can develop anywhere.

The only way to eliminate neurodermatitis is to break the itch-scratch cycle:

☐ Don't wear irritating fabrics such as wool, silk, or rough synthetics. Instead, try to wear absorbent, nonirritating materials next to the skin.

☐ To suppress the urge to scratch, apply an ice-cold compress.

☐ You might want to apply an over-the-counter hydrocortisone cream (*Cortaid*) and cover with a bandage. (But don't use such drugs for longer than two to three weeks, since they can thin the skin.)

☐ If itching makes it hard for you to fall asleep, try an over-the-counter antihistamine such as diphenhydramine *(Benadryl)*. A simple over-the-counter pain reliever—aspirin, acetaminophen *(Tylenol)*, or ibuprofen *(Advil)*—can also bring relief.

☐ Since many sufferers scratch when they're asleep, keep your fingernails short.

Where There's a Rash

A widespread itchy rash indicates other problems. Sometimes, an allergic reaction to a certain food or medication will lead to a sudden bout of hives—a raised red rash that spreads over the body and itches like crazy. Although such a reaction usually occurs within just a few hours after ingesting the offending food or drug, it can take as long as a week to show up after a final dose of certain antibiotics, including penicillin. Many times, expert detective work is needed to track down the culprit.

In addition to things that you ingest, things that you touch can also make you itch. Contact dermatitis can be brought on by plants, cosmetics, chemicals, even rough clothing and harsh soaps or laundry detergents. Hours or possibly days after contact, a very itchy, red, blistery rash develops. Again, the trick is to identify and avoid the offending item.

Silvery, scaly patches are a sure sign of psoriasis. While the condition commonly occurs on the elbows or knees, it can also affect the entire body, including the scalp. The rash isn't always itchy, but it can be—very. Psoriasis usually clears temporarily in response to ultraviolet light, either from sunlight or a special lamp. If there are only small patches, a hydrocortisone cream can help. Or your doctor may prescribe a more potent corticosteroid cream.

Itching All Over

When there's no sign of a rash, itching "all over" can be a symptom of an internal disorder. Such itching can signal diseases of the liver, kidneys, or thyroid gland. If lab tests detect such a disease, proper treatment can resolve the itch as well.

By far the most common cause of generalized itching without a noticeable rash is simply dry skin. As you age, your skin thins and oil glands produce less of a protective barrier on the skin surface. This leaves your skin more vulnerable to minor irritations. The problem is especially severe in wintertime, when humidity is low.

Fortunately, there are several ways you can protect your skin:

- ☐ To preserve your natural protective oils, take shorter and less frequent baths or showers, and use lukewarm water.
- ☐ Use a mild soap—one that's low in alkaline, such as *Dove* or *Neutrogena*. Apply the soap only to your face, armpits, genital and anal areas, and hands and feet.
- ☐ If you bathe rather than shower, add a little water-dispersible bath oil, such as *Alpha Keri*. (Be sure to use a rubber mat in the tub to avoid slipping.)
- ☐ Immediately after bathing, apply bath oil to your moist skin. Avoid alcohol-containing lotions, which dry out the skin.
- ☐ Don't air-dry after bathing; that tends to chap your skin. Pat dry with an absorbent towel.
- ☐ Use a room humidifier during winter.
- ☐ Keep room temperatures on the cool side, since warmth can worsen an itch.
- ☐ In cold weather, wear gloves and a scarf or ski mask to limit the evaporation of moisture from your hands and face.
- ☐ Use a mild laundry detergent—one that has no enzymes or perfumes, such as *Cheerfree* or *Ecover*. Rinse clothes well.

☐ OFFICE VISIT

Fingernail Facts and Fallacies

An 18-year-old high school senior came to see me for her precollege physical exam. She said she wanted to talk about something but felt embarrassed. Anticipating a discussion of birth-control methods, I encouraged her to go on.

"What can I do about my nails?" she asked. "They break for no reason at all."

As we talked, I found a very good reason. For the past two years, she'd been on the varsity swim team. The water had weakened her nails to the breaking point. It turned out that she wasn't planning to join the swim team in college. Within a few months, her nails were back to normal.

It's not just swimmers who have brittle fingernails. In fact, nail weakness is among the most common medical complaints. And sometimes nail problems can provide clues to the presence of serious disease.

Deformity and Disease

Nails often have bumps and other flaws that don't signal any problem. Vertical ridges become more common and usually more pronounced as people age. White lines and tiny white spots are common, too.

Occasionally, however, unusual nail features do reflect disease. For that reason, physicians often examine your fingernails along with the rest of you. Here are some possible fingernail clues:

☐ Deformities such as pitting, spooning (in which the nail curls upward), and separation of the nail from its bed can be caused by diseases as diverse as psoriasis, anemia, and hypothyroidism.

☐ Nail color can also indicate disease, since nails are usually a healthy pink. Pale or whitish nails, for example, suggest anemia; bluish nails, caused by insufficient oxygen in the blood, could mean poisoning, heart failure, or chronic lung trouble.

☐ Thick, distorted fingernails can be caused by a fungal infection.

☐ Rounding and expansion of both the nails and the end of the fingers, which may become clublike, can reflect a variety of serious conditions, ranging from lung cancer to inflammatory bowel disease.

☐ A horizontal furrow, called a "beau's line," can result from major surgery, heart attack, or other serious illness, any of which can slow nail growth abruptly. The line eventually grows out.

Wear and Tear

A number of diseases, such as an overactive thyroid gland and anemia, can make nails brittle. Usually, though, nails weaken simply because they're subjected to so much everyday abuse.

Take water, for example—the most common cause of brittle nails. While fingernails may feel hard and look waterproof, they're actually highly permeable. As nails absorb water, they swell; when they dry, they shrink. Repeat that cycle often enough—particularly in cold, dry weather, which already dries the nails—and they'll break or split at the ends.

Solvents, such as those in household cleaners, can also penetrate and chemically dry the nails. And activities like gardening and sports can break unprotected nails.

What passes for "nail care" can be a form of abuse. Various products, such as polish removers, can weaken the nails. An overly aggressive manicure can damage the nails. Worse, it can damage the cuticle, allowing infection to develop under the nail.

Proper Care

Here are some basic suggestions that will help to ensure the health of your fingernails:

☐ Protect your nails from the ravages of water. Wear cotton-lined rubber gloves when doing household chores such as washing dishes.

☐ Immediately after exposure to water, apply an ordinary moisturizing lotion to your nails as well as your hands.

☐ Wear gloves in cold weather and during activities that might harm your nails.

☐ Keep your nails short to help prevent breakage. Before trimming, soak them in water for a few minutes so they'll be less brittle under the clipper. File only in one direction—not back and forth, which can create splits. Apply moisturizer afterward.

☐ Don't pick at hangnails; that can break the skin and invite infection. Clip hangnails off close to the skin surface with sharp cuticle scissors.

- Avoid nail polish removers that contain acetone, which can dry nails; look for products that contain acetate instead. And use any remover as infrequently as possible.
- Don't waste your money on vitamins, calcium, or gelatin. No supplements will improve the way your nails grow.

Stuttering

Hotline for Stuttering

Q. *I started stuttering about three years ago, and it's getting worse. The problem is especially severe during job interviews or when I make a speech. Where can I get help?*

A. Your stuttering very possibly began in your childhood, without your being aware of it. Recent stress may have made a preexisting problem more noticeable. Speech therapists now offer a number of techniques that can improve fluency for most stutterers. To find out about speech clinics and qualified speech therapists in your area, call the American Speech-Language-Hearing Association's toll-free number, 800-638-8255, weekdays from 10:00 A.M. to 4:00 P.M., eastern standard time.

Sweating Problems

Night Sweats

Q. *For almost two years, I've sweated heavily at night. Some nights I have to change my pajamas twice or even change the sheets. My family doctor as well as a cardiologist and a neurologist have found nothing wrong with me. I'm a 74-year-old man. What could be causing the problem?*

A. Sometimes it's hard to pinpoint the cause of recurrent night sweats. Your doctors have probably ruled out the serious causes, such as chronic infections and certain malignant tumors. Use of alcohol or over-the-counter pain relievers (aspirin, acetaminophen, or ibuprofen) before bedtime can also make you sweat. Sometimes sweating accompanies the normal drop in body temperature at night; that can be a major nuisance, but it's not harmful.

☐ OFFICE VISIT

Breaking Out of a Heavy Sweat

"It's not just embarrassing—it could cost me my job."

A distressed young salesman was telling me about a problem that had plagued him since his college years: He sweated heavily, especially from his underarms. In fact, I had already noticed.

"At first, it happened only in tough situations like taking an important exam or going out on a first date," he confided. "But it got worse, and now it happens anytime, sometimes all day long. I keep having to leave business meetings because my shirt and jacket are soaked. I'm lucky I live close to my office—I have to go home and shower four times a day."

This man had one of the worst problems with sweating I'd ever seen. He clearly needed medical help. But people with a more moderate problem can take steps to control the sweating on their own.

Perspiration Information

Ordinarily, the sweat glands start working when body temperature rises, usually due to exercise or exposure to heat. The sweat glands also respond to emotional stress, such as nervousness, embarrassment, or sexual excitement.

When there's no source of heat or emotion, sweating can result from menopausal flushes or simply from being overweight. It can also follow a hot, spicy meal. In some cases, abnormal sweating indicates an underlying disorder, such as infection, an overactive thyroid, certain endocrine or chest tumors, nerve inflammation, tuberculosis, or Hodgkin's disease.

My patient, however, had a clean bill of health and wasn't an especially emotional man. Like other people who sweat too much, his sweating mechanism just took off on its own and wreaked havoc with his life.

Self-Treatment Strategies

If you're troubled by underarm sweating, try these measures first:

☐ Make sure you're using an antiperspirant, not just a plain deodorant. Deodorants may contain fragrances, antibacterials, and absorbent powders. Antiperspirants may have all of those things, but they also contain aluminum salts, which block the ducts of the sweat glands.

☐ If the antiperspirant you're using doesn't help, try another. Different people respond differently to the various formulations on the market. In general, roll-ons and sticks give the most protection; aerosols and other sprays, the least.

☐ For best results, apply the antiperspirant long before you need it, perhaps as early as the night before—even if you'll be showering when you get up. Then reapply in the morning. It can take several hours—and sometimes repeated applications over several days—for the stuff to become fully effective.

☐ Before applying a liquid roll-on or an antiperspirant, shake it to stir up active ingredients that may have settled to the bottom.

☐ Be sure to dry yourself thoroughly before applying an antiperspirant, since moisture dilutes the ingredients. Don't bother applying it once you're sweating; it won't work at all.

□ Wear loose-fitting, natural fabrics such as cotton and linen, which are more absorbent than synthetic fabrics. Natural fibers also allow perspiration to evaporate.

No Sweat

For people who sweat extra heavily, such self-help measures can't stem the flow; medical intervention is almost always necessary.

The first step is to try a strong antiperspirant available only by prescription. *Drysol* contains 20 percent aluminum chloride hexa-hydrate, which is many times more concentrated than the aluminum salts used in regular commercial products. You don't apply *Drysol* in the usual way; you spread it on before going to bed, keep the area covered overnight with a plastic-wrap dressing, and wash it off in the morning. Most people get by with one to three applications per week, at roughly 25 cents a shot. Others must keep reapplying *Drysol* every night, provided they don't develop a skin rash.

When prescription antiperspirants are not enough, the next step might be to try a technique called iontophoresis—the application of a weak electric current to the problem area. There's no pain, just a mild tingling sensation. Typically, a dermatologist trains you to operate the device, which you then use at home for 20 minutes or so a day. After 10 to 14 days, one treatment a week may be enough to keep sweating under control. The device costs about $750, including the professional training sessions.

A similar device called the *Drionic* is now available without a prescription from General Medical Company in Los Angeles. At $125, it's much cheaper than the prescription unit. But since the current is weaker, some experts believe that it may not be as effective in particularly severe cases.

Many medications have been tried for severe sweating. The two current options are propantheline *(Pro-Banthīne)*, typically used to treat intestinal spasms, and propranolol *(Inderal)*, usually used for hypertension. But these drugs don't always help and they can have side effects, ranging from dry mouth to drowsiness to slowing of the heart rate. So the dosage must be modified to suit the individual and monitored periodically. Depending on the drug and the dosage, treatment can cost anywhere from $10 to $80 a month.

If one or another of these measures and the passage of time fail to bring relief, surgery to remove the underarm sweat glands may be justified. (You can get along fine without them.) The operation is done under general anesthesia, takes two to three hours, and costs about $2,500.

Recently, physicians have started using a simpler, safer method: liposuction. A plastic surgeon or dermatologist removes the sweat glands by suction through a tube, so the incision and resulting scar are much smaller. The operation is usually done on an outpatient basis under local anesthesia and takes about an hour or two. Since this is a new application for liposuction, it's important to find a practitioner who's experienced in the technique. The cost ranges from $2,000 to $3,000, which should be covered by health insurance. However, your doctor must let the insurer know that it was done for medical, not cosmetic, purposes.

The Thyroid

Thyroid and Decongestants

Q. *I've been taking thyroid hormone for about 10 years. Recently, I've noticed that cold remedies containing a decongestant now include a warning not to take them if you have thyroid disease. Does that mean I should stop taking those remedies?*

A. Only if they cause annoying side effects, such as nervousness, insomnia, or heart "palpitations". In that case, switch to a topical decongestant, such as 0.5 percent phenylephrine (*Neo-Synephrine*), which doesn't interact with thyroid medication.

Hypothyroidism or Laziness?

Q. *I used to be tired all the time, until doctors diagnosed a thyroid tumor. Before removing it, they started me on thyroid-hormone pills, which I continue to take every day. Almost immediately, my fatigue disappeared and hasn't returned. Is it possible that many people who are considered lazy actually have hypothyroidism?*

A. Not likely. Thirty or so years ago, thyroid hormone was the fashionable treatment for unexplained lethargy. Many people were unnecessarily "pepped up" with thyroid-hormone pills for years, often without a proper diagnosis of hypothyroidism (underactive thyroid gland). Today we know that hypothyroidism is not a common cause of chronic fatigue alone. There are usually other symptoms of hypothyroidism, including coarse scalp hair, intolerance to cold temperatures, constipation, dry skin, hoarseness, muscle cramps, and weight gain.

Long-Term Thyroid Therapy

Q. *In 1950 I was placed on thyroid-hormone therapy, and I've been taking 2 grains a day ever since. What are the likely consequences of such long-term medication?*

A. Assuming hypothyroidism was properly diagnosed in the first place, the medication is replacing what your own thyroid can't make. The adequacy of that dose can be verified by having your physician order a serum TSH (thyroid-stimulating hormone) level. Suppression of serum TSH below the normal range for many years can cause bone loss (osteoporosis), which could make you more vulnerable to fracture.

Thyroid Pill Dependency?

Q. *I've taken a small dose of thyroid hormone every day for 40 years. My doctor hadn't diagnosed hypothyroidism; he just recommended the medication for chronic fatigue. Should I stop taking it?*

A. Probably. However, even though you may not have really needed the drug initially, your thyroid gland has adjusted to the supplement by decreasing its normal production of thyroid hormone. So if you go off the drug now, your thyroid gland could take up to six weeks to recover and you might suffer temporary symptoms of hypothyroidism, such as weight gain and sluggishness.

Still, it's better to avoid medication when your body can do the job itself. If you're willing to put up with those symptoms for a few weeks, talk to your physician about discontinuing the pills.

Underactive Thyroid?

Q. *According to information in a popular medical book, I may have an underactive thyroid gland. My hair, skin, eyes, and mouth are very dry; I have puffiness under my eyes, and I'm very sensitive to cold on my back. But a blood test indicates my thyroid is normal. Are there other ways I should be tested for an underactive thyroid?*

A. Not if you've had the two appropriate blood tests. One measures thyroid hormone itself, and one measures thyroid-stimulating hormone, or TSH. Your symptoms could be caused by many other problems, including dry environment, medical conditions that dry out the eyes, and certain skin diseases.

☐ Tuberculosis

Wary of TB Drug

Q. *I'm a healthy 28-year-old woman. After a positive tuberculosis skin test (but a negative chest X ray), my physician prescribed 300 milligrams a day of INH for nine months. I've been told the drug can cause hepatitis and must be carefully monitored. Liver tests at three months* *were normal, but I'm still insecure about the possibility of hepatitis during this long-term therapy. What do you recommend?*

A. Complete the prescribed therapy, and continue to be monitored monthly. Isoniazid (INH) is highly effective in preventing the development of active tuberculosis in people with positive skin tests. The risk of drug-induced liver inflammation, or "chemical" hepatitis, is low at your age. But it increases with age and alcohol consumption, and after age 35, the risk becomes greater than that of developing tuberculosis. Accordingly, the drug is not recommended after 35 unless the person is a "recent converter"—someone who had a negative skin test within the last year or two but then tested positive. Liver problems, if they occur at all, usually appear within the first four months of treatment. If liver function tests show abnormal results, stopping the drug generally results in complete recovery from "chemical" hepatitis.

☐ Water: Diet and Safety

How Much Water?

Q. *I've heard you should drink eight glasses of water a day. Must I?*

A. Not if you don't want to. The body does require about 1 to 2 quarts of water a day, which equals four to eight 8-ounce glasses. But that doesn't mean you have to drink that much water. You also get water from foods and from other beverages. Usually, all you need to do is drink when you're thirsty. More attention to water is necessary when diarrhea, diuretic medications, extreme heat, strenuous activity, vomiting, or anything else is causing excessive fluid loss.

Mineral Water Safety

Q. *The label on my brand of mineral water states: "Like other mineral waters, this should not be used as a sole source of drinking water." Is it safe to drink mineral water?*

A. Yes, but not liberally. Unlike bottled still water, mineral water is not tested and regulated by the FDA. Most mineral waters contain dissolved solids, sometimes even small amounts of toxic minerals such as arsenic. A daily glass or two shouldn't hurt you; but, as the label states, mineral water should not be your sole source of drinking water.

Water and Dieting

Q. *Some diet programs have you drink 10 glasses of water a day. What's the point?*

A. The main reason is to prevent kidney stones. Very-low-calorie diet programs can break down the body's protein stores, resulting in excess uric acid in the blood. When excreted in the urine, the excess acid can lead to kidney stones. Drinking large quantities of fluids dilutes the urine and lessens the likelihood of stones. In addition, drinking water frequently can stop hunger contractions of the stomach and create a temporary sensation of fullness.

Well-Water Safety

Q. *We recently moved to the country. Is well water automatically better for my family than city water, or can it be just as dangerous? Also, now that we're not drinking fluoridated water, what should I do to keep my family's teeth healthy?*

A. Well water is by no means automatically safer than city water. In fact, for well-run city systems supplied by protected reservoirs, the reverse may be true.

The quality of well water depends on what's in the underground aquifer from which it's drawn. Among potential aquifer pollutants are septic tank seepage, gasoline from leaking underground tanks, agricultural fertilizers and pesticides, road salt, and industrial wastes. To make certain your well is safe, have the water tested by a reputable laboratory. Your state health department might test your water for you, or suggest a lab to do so. Also check with your local water authority to determine whether periodic testing is advisable.

Make sure the initial test covers fluoride, which occurs naturally in some well water. Children under 14 need fluoride to strengthen their developing teeth. If your water doesn't have the optimal amount, your dentist or pediatrician can prescribe drops or chewable tablets. Using fluoridated toothpaste and fluoride rinses is sufficient to protect against tooth decay in most teenagers and adults.

☐ Weight Control

Can Diet Sodas Add Weight?

Q. *I know diet sodas have few or no calories. But I seem to gain weight when I drink them. Could that be because they contain more sodium than regular soda and make me retain fluids?*

A. Diet soda isn't what's making you gain weight. That comes from eating too much or exercising too little. Many diet sodas do have more sodium than regular soda does. A 12-ounce can of *Diet 7-Up*, for example, contains about 70 milligrams of sodium, whereas regular *7-Up* has 32 milligrams.

But 70 milligrams isn't a lot. Since Americans consume about 2,300 to 6,900 milligrams of sodium a day, you'd have to guzzle lots of diet pop to boost your sodium intake significantly. Even if you did drink so much, the sodium wouldn't make your body retain a noticeable amount of fluid unless you had heart or kidney problems. People on sodium-restricted diets, however, probably shouldn't drink more than one or two cans of soda a day.

Flabby Abdomen

Q. *How can a person lose fat from the lower abdomen when the rest of the body is relatively lean?*

A. As we've pointed out before, there's no such thing as "spot reduction" exercises that zero in on fat in a specific area. When you work out, you use energy produced by burning fat from all over your body—not just around the muscles doing the most work. So aside from burning a few calories, all that exercises such as sit-ups do is strengthen your abdominal muscles and help hold your gut in.

However, studies do suggest that people losing weight—whether through any sort of exercise, calorie reduction, or both—tend to shed abdominal fat faster than fat from other parts of the body. That's good news, not only for your appearance, but also for your health: Abdominal fat seems to pose a higher risk of coronary heart disease than fat deposited in other areas.

Middle-Age Spread

Q. *What is the best way to control middle-age spread: diet, exercise, or both?*

A. Both—including exercises to tone muscles and burn fat.

People acquire body fat in two distinct patterns. In so-called middle-age spread, fat accumulates in a "spare tire" around the belly, giving you an apple shape. The other distribution is pear-shaped, with fat deposited around the hips rather than the waist. Men are most often "apples"; women, most often "pears."

Exercises that strengthen your stomach muscles, such as sit-ups, can help restrain a bulging belly. But they won't reduce the amount of abdominal fat. The only way to take that fat off and keep it off is to eat fewer calories and do exercises like biking, jogging, swimming, and walking, which burn a lot of calories.

Skinny People, Fatty Diet

Q. *Since I'm very thin and want to gain weight, I eat plenty of fatty foods. Will my low weight keep my blood-cholesterol levels down despite the high-fat diet?*

A. No. A high-fat diet can increase blood-cholesterol levels in thin people as well as in heavy people. The body's tendency to convert dietary fat into blood cholesterol is entirely separate from its tendency to deposit that fat on your waist or thighs. To try to gain weight, increase your consumption of a variety of foods, not just fatty ones. But remember that thin people can have just as much trouble gaining weight and keeping it on as most heavy people do losing weight and keeping it off.

Why Thin People Don't Gain

Q. *Why do some people stay too thin even though they're trying to gain weight?*

A. Like their heavy counterparts, thin people seem to be programmed to remain close to a certain weight. They might be able to add pounds by cultivating patently unhealthy habits—avoiding exercise and gorging on high-calorie foods. But most thin people who tried to live that dieter's dream would actually find it hard to stay underactive and overindulgent. Eventually, they'd revert to their usual habits and usual weight.

Thin people do have another option: muscle-building exercises. But again, the extra weight will be lost if they stop pumping iron.

Women's Health

Annual Pap Smear

Q. *How often should a woman get a Pap smear? And what time of month gives the most accurate results?*

A. The venerable Pap smear is one of the most important cancer-detection tests. A woman should begin having an annual Pap smear at age 18 (or earlier, if she is sexually active). Some gynecologists recommend that women at high risk for cervical cancer be tested even more frequently. (Risk factors include multiple sex partners, herpes simplex virus type 2 infection, and venereal warts.)

Pap smears should not be done during the menstrual period. Some recent data suggest that the test is more accurate during the first half of the cycle, if you use oral contraceptives. Midcycle is preferred for most other menstruating women.

Regardless of when the test is done, the technician reading the smear must know if you're taking oral contraceptives or estrogen replacement therapy, as well as when your last menstrual period began. Only with this information can the smear be accurately interpreted.

Antibiotics and Yeast

Q. *Every time I take antibiotics, I end up with a yeast infection. How can I prevent this?*

A. Whether or not yeast infections can be prevented is a matter of controversy. Since you always seem to get an infection when taking antibiotics, you could try using an antifungal vaginal cream at the same time. These creams include clotrimazole (*Femcare,*

Gyne-Lotrimin) and miconazole (*Monistat*), sold over the counter. Another product, butoconazole (*Femstat*), is available by prescription.

Breast Tenderness

Q. *For breast tenderness, my gynecologist recommended 1,200 IU of vitamin E a day for life. He also recommended cutting back on caffeine. Are those treatments effective?*

A. There's no convincing evidence that eliminating caffeine or adding vitamin E helps relieve breast pain, which is usually caused by fluid retained just before menstruation. If your pain does precede menstruation, you might try taking a mild diuretic during the few days before your period. An over-the-counter pain reliever and a supportive bra might also help.

Breast-feeding and Cancer

Q. *I've read that some studies suggest that breast-feeding reduces a woman's risk of developing breast cancer. What's the current thinking on this?*

A. Most of the evidence hints at only a weak association at best. And at least one research team has found another explanation for the slightly lower rate of cancer among women who have breast-fed: Women who cannot produce enough milk to breast-feed seem to have a slightly higher risk of developing breast cancer to begin with. Overall, a woman's chance of getting breast cancer appears to be about the same whether or not she's ever breast-fed a baby.

Concern About Abnormal Pap Tests

Q. *My Pap tests have shown "slightly abnormal" cells for nearly two years now. Other than recommending more frequent testing, my doctors* have not suggested any treatment. Recently I read in a newspaper column that "aggressive treatment" is necessary for premalignant stages of cervical neoplasia. What do you recommend?

A. Although "slightly abnormal" changes are not necessarily premalignant, Consumers Union's medical consultants nonetheless recommend that you seek another opinion. Reasons for an abnormal Pap test result can range from vaginal or cervical infection to true cancer of the cervix. If the cause is an infection, treatment will usually lead to a normal Pap test; if not, the abnormality should be investigated further.

Estrogen After Hysterectomy

Q. I was grateful for your information on estrogen and progestin replacement for women approaching menopause. However, you included no information for young women who have had to undergo a complete hysterectomy. Four years ago, at age 30, I went through this operation. After taking estrogen in several forms, I continue to have severe mood swings, hot flashes, depression, severe headaches, nervous conditions, and sharp pains in both of my breasts. Help!

A. Your persistent hot flashes suggest that your dose of estrogen may be too low. Young women who have had a hysterectomy sometimes need more estrogen than older women going through menopause, in order to relieve the uncomfortable symptoms of abrupt hormonal decline. Your physician should work with you to find the dosage that is most effective.

Estrogen Cream: How Safe?

Q. Would you comment on the possible adverse effects of estrogen in creams prescribed to treat vaginal dryness in postmenopausal women? Do they pose a risk to women with a family history of cancer?

A. The risk is minimal. Although estrogen from these creams is absorbed into the bloodstream, no study to date has shown a health hazard from the use of vaginal estrogens. Most women will need to use the creams only about twice a week, which should be safe even if a woman has a family history of cancer. A woman who has had uterine or breast cancer herself, however, should not use estrogen in any form.

Estrogen: Why Not Generic?

Q. *Why has the manufacture of generic estrogen been discontinued, forcing us to pay almost four times as much for* Premarin?

A. The FDA tells us that makers of generic conjugated estrogens have failed to prove their products are absorbed into the blood-stream in the same way—and at the same rate—as brand-name estrogens.

Hot Flashes and Diuretics

Q. *I've heard that the water-ridding properties of diuretics such as* Dyazide *[triamterene/hydrochlorothiazide] make it essential to drink plenty of fluids during hot weather to prevent dehydration. Since the hot flashes that accompany menopause can also make you sweat, would that likewise lead to a dehydration risk from diuretics?*

A. No. Menopausal hot flashes are caused by temporarily dilated blood vessels. While that may make you sweat, you won't lose a significant amount of water, even if you're taking a diuretic.

Hunched Back

Q. *I'm a 63-year-old woman and am starting to develop a hunched back. Is there some exercise to delay that?*

A. No. Your problem is probably osteoporosis, or bone thinning, which commonly follows menopause. The weakened spinal vertebrae simply fracture and collapse. You should consult your physician about the treatment options for osteoporosis, which include taking the female hormone estrogen (*Premarin*), the injectable hormone calcitonin (*Calcimar*), and the drug etidronate (*Didronel*).

Illicit Drugs: Pregnancy Peril?

Q. *Ten years ago, in college, I experimented with several drugs, including marijuana, cocaine, and LSD. Now I'm 30 and my husband and I are thinking about starting a family. Have I done any permanent damage to my egg supply? Is the risk of birth defects increased?*

A. Go ahead and start your family. With the exception of certain anticancer medications, prior drug use, by males or females, has no known lasting effects on reproduction.

Nystatin for Yeast "Allergy"

Q. *In your report on yeast allergy, you called both the disorder and the remedies phony. That's got me worried. A holistic doctor has me taking nystatin because of a yeast allergy. Have I been had?*

A. Afraid so. Nystatin is a perfectly legitimate drug for proven infections due to candida, a yeast. But for nonexistent disorders such as yeast allergy, legitimate drugs are no better than fakes.

Osteoporosis and the Pill

Q. *From age 18 to 26 I had no menstrual periods. When my gynecologist prescribed birth-control pills a year ago, my menstrual cycle resumed. I've heard that lack of periods increases the risk of osteoporosis. Since birth-control pills contain estrogen, will they help reduce my risk?*

A. In your case, yes. Amenorrhea (the absence of periods) is usually associated with decreased production of the female hormone estrogen by the ovaries. Lack of estrogen can eventually lead to osteoporosis, which is characterized by less dense—and thus more fragile—bones. The birth-control pills are providing you with estrogen and helping prevent further bone loss. Women with normal periods already produce all the estrogen they need, so the Pill makes no difference to them.

An adequate calcium intake (at least 1,000 milligrams a day) and regular weight-bearing exercise before menopause can help build bone mass and protect against the chance of postmenopausal osteoporosis.

Ovarian Cancer Clue?

Q. *I have heard on two television talk shows about a screening test for early diagnosis of ovarian cancer. What is the test and is it effective?*

A. A blood test called CA-125 is being used to monitor the treatment of women with ovarian cancer, and to check for recurrence. The test is very sensitive but not specific: It can detect ovarian cancer, but it also can turn up positive in the presence of other conditions, including pregnancy, endometriosis, uterine fibroids, and pelvic inflammatory disease. For that reason, many physicians do not use CA-125 as a screening test for ovarian cancer unless a woman is at high risk because of family history. These women should have a CA-125 blood test annually, and should discuss with their physician the suitability of having an annual ultrasound examination of the ovaries.

Pap Tests and Medicare

Q. *Medicare has rejected my insurance claim for a routine Pap smear. Is this standard Medicare policy?*

A. Until a few years ago, Medicare did not provide a reimbursement for routine screening procedures. Only medical services prompted by illness or injury were covered. However, Medicare now reimburses patients for a routine screening Pap test once every three years. While this is a change in the right direction, it still won't provide coverage for the annual Pap smear recommended by Consumers Union's medical consultants. And, for women at high risk for cervical cancer, some gynecologists recommend even more frequent testing.

Postpartum Depression

Q. *What causes postpartum depression? What are the latest treatments?*

A. Postpartum depression—not the more common postpartum "blues"—is a psychiatric disorder that can severely impair day-to-day functioning. Its onset is usually within the first few weeks or months after childbirth. A woman who has once had postpartum depression can experience it again after future births.

The causes of postpartum depression are not well understood. The sudden change from the pregnant state, with accompanying changes in hormone levels, probably plays some role.

In contrast to the self-limited "blues," which usually lasts only a short time and needs only emotional support, true postpartum depression requires the attention of a psychiatrist. Antidepressant medications can help. Rarely, electroconvulsive (electric shock) therapy may be necessary.

Shrinking Fibroids

Q. *I have several uterine fibroids but would like to avoid a hysterectomy. I've been told that daily injections of Lupron or monthly injections of Lupron Depot will shrink fibroids. Are these medications safe?*

Since estrogen causes fibroids to grow, should I avoid meat, poultry, and alcohol, which, I have read, contain estrogen?

A. Fibroids are benign growths of the uterus. Depending on their size, they may cause excessive menstrual bleeding and pressure on pelvic organs, or no symptoms at all. Fibroids usually shrink at menopause, when estrogen levels decline.

The drugs you mention act on the pituitary gland and shrink fibroids by decreasing the amount of estrogen secreted by the ovaries. Both drugs are safe, but they can produce menopausal symptoms such as flushes, sweats, and mood swings. They are also very expensive.

Cattle (not poultry) are given estrogen to promote growth, but the residues in meat, if any, are too small to affect the human body. Naturally occurring plant estrogens have been identified in bourbon and beer; again, however, the quantities present are unlikely to affect fibroid size.

Time out from the Pill?

Q. *My doctor recommended that I stop taking birth-control pills for three months every three years so they don't affect my chance of conceiving when I'm ready. What evidence is there to support her claim?*

A. None at all. That was a concern when the Pill was first introduced, but not anymore. Most women resume normal ovulatory cycles immediately after the Pill is stopped, no matter how long they've been on it. Occasionally, the first post-Pill cycle may occur without ovulation. In rare instances—usually in women who've had irregular menstrual periods prior to using the Pill—the delay may last several months or more. There is no harm in attempting to conceive immediately after discontinuing the Pill.

Index